P9-CFN-661

Review of Organic Functional Groups

Introduction to Medicinal Organic Chemistry

Review of Organic Functional Groups

Introduction to Medicinal Organic Chemistry

Fourth Edition

Thomas L. Lemke, PhD
Associate Dean for Administration and
Professor of Medicinal Chemistry
College of Pharmacy
University of Houston
Houston, Texas

Editor: David B. Troy
Managing Editor: Matthew J. Hauber
Marketing Manager: Samantha Smith
Production Editor: Jennifer Ajello
Designer: Doug Smock
Compositor: Maryland Composition
Printer: R.R. Donnelly & Sons-Crawfordsville

Copyright © 2003 Lippincott Williams & Wilkins

351 West Camden Street
Baltimore, MD 21201

530 Walnut Street
Philadelphia, PA 19106

All rights reserved. This book is protected by copyright. No part of this book may be reproduced in any form or by any means, including photocopying, or utilized by any information storage and retrieval system without written permission from the copyright owner.

The publisher is not responsible (as a matter of product liability, negligence, or otherwise) for any injury resulting from any material contained herein. This publication contains information relating to general principles of medical care that should not be construed as specific instructions for individual patients. Manufacturers' product information and package inserts should be reviewed for current information, including contraindications, dosages, and precautions.

Printed in the United States of America

First Edition, 1983
Second Edition, 1987
Third Edition, 1992

Library of Congress Cataloging-in-Publication Data

Lemke, Thomas L.
  Review of organic functional groups: introduction to medicinal organic chemistry/
Thomas L. Lemke.—4th ed.
    p.; cm.
  Includes index.
  ISBN 0-7817-4381-8
  1. Pharmaceutical chemistry. 2. Chemistry, Organic. I. Title.
  [DNLM: 1. Chemistry, Organic. 2. Chemistry, Pharmaceutical. QV 744 L554r 2003]
RS403.L397 2003
615'3—dc21

                                                                    2003051692

The publishers have made every effort to trace the copyright holders for borrowed material. If they have inadvertently overlooked any, they will be pleased to make the necessary arrangements at the first opportunity.

To purchase additional copies of this book, call our customer service department at **(800) 638-3030** or fax orders to **(301) 824-7390.** International customers should call **(301) 714-2324.**

Visit Lippincott Williams & Wilkins on the Internet: http://www.LWW.com. Lippincott Williams & Wilkins customer service representatives are available from 8:30 am to 6:00 pm, EST.

04 05 06 07 08
2 3 4 5 6 7 8 9 10

Introduction

This book has been prepared with the intent that it may be used as a self-paced review of organic functional groups. If the material covered in this book were to be presented in a conventional classroom setting, it would require 14 to 16 formal lecture hours. With this in mind, you should not attempt to cover all of the material in one sitting. A slow, leisurely pace will greatly increase your comprehension and decrease the number of return visits to the material. You should stop to review any section that you do not completely understand. Added to this edition of the book is an electronic set of questions designed around each chapter. The questions are followed by a detailed explanation of the correct answer. Enclosed with this book is an Electronic Workbook CD-Rom composed of problem sets corresponding to each of the organic functional groups (Chapters 2–15 and 17). Each problem set is followed by answers to the questions and a detailed discussion explaining the process leading to the answers. If you do not understand an answer or the process leading to the answer, return to the appropriate section of the book and review that section again.

OBJECTIVES

The following outline is a general review of the functional groups common to organic chemistry. It is the objective of this book to review the general topics of nomenclature, physical properties (with specific emphasis placed on water and lipid solubility), chemical properties (the stability or lack of stability of a functional group to normal environmental conditions, referred to as in vitro stability), and metabolism (the stability of lack of stability of a functional group in the body, referred to as in vivo stability). There will be no attempt to cover synthesis, nor will great emphasis be placed on chemical reactions except when they related to the physical or chemical stability and mechanistic action of drugs. This review is meant to provide background material for the formal pharmacy courses in medicinal chemistry. The objectives are presented in the following manner to aid in focusing attention on the expected learning outcomes.

Upon successful completion of the book, the following goals will have been attained:

- The student will be able to draw a chemical structure of simple organic molecules given a common or official chemical name. With more complex polyfunctional molecules, the student will be able to identify the functional groups given the chemical structure.

- The student will be able to predict the solubility of a chemical in:
  1. Aqueous acid
  2. Water
  3. Aqueous base
- The student will be able to predict and show, with chemical structures, the chemical instabilities of each organic functional group under conditions appropriate to a substance "setting on the shelf," by which is meant conditions such as air, light, aqueous acid or base, and heat.
- The student will be able to predict and show, with chemical structures, the metabolism of each organic functional group.

To help you master these skills, the information is presented in the following order:

- *Nomenclature*
  1. Common
  2. Official (IUPAC)
- *Physical-Chemical Properties*
  1. Physical properties—related to water and lipid solubility
  2. Chemical properties in vitro—stability or reactivity of functional groups "on the shelf"
- *Metabolism*
  Chemical properties in vivo—stability or reactivity of functional groups "in the body"

RECOMMENDED PREPARATION

To maximize learning and to provide perspective in the study of the book, it would be helpful to read certain background material. It is highly recommended that a textbook on general organic chemistry be reviewed and consulted as a reference book while using this book. Pay special attention to the sections on nomenclature and physical-chemical properties.

Acknowledgments

This book would not have been possible without the encouragement and input of colleagues at my own institution and from medicinal chemists throughout the United States. The idea for the text originated from a late night discussion at a Medicinal Symposium but came to fruition because of support from SmithKline Corporation and students at the University of Houston College of Pharmacy. Continuous suggestions have come from those faculty who actually make use of the book and this has led to the changes which are found in previous editions as well as this edition of the book. I would especially like to thank Dr. Louis Williams for his timely comments. And the real joy comes from students, some of whom are now my colleagues, who informally tell me of the benefits they have gained from this book.

I must also acknowledge the excellent staff, past and present, at LWW who have made this project seem more like an academic undertaking rather than a commercial process. Many of the staff members I have only met electronically or via phone conversations, but their contributions have led to a more readable text. I would like to specifically acknowledge Donna Balado for her past support and David B. Troy for making this edition happen. The continuous support at LWW has come from managing editor Matthew J. Hauber. Without Matt's problem-solving ability and encouragement, I am certain that this edition would have been a labor of work rather than joy. Finally, a very special thank you to my wife Pat for putting up with the hours of time put into the text.

T.L.L.

Contents

Water Solubility and Chemical Bonding

At the outset, several definitions relating to organic compounds need to be discussed.

For our purposes, we will assume that an organic molecule will dissolve either in water or in a nonaqueous lipid solvent; that is, the organic molecule will not remain undissolved at the interphase of water and a lipid solvent. If a molecule dissolves fully or partially in water, it is said to be hydrophilic or to have hydrophilic character. The word "hydrophilic" is derived from "hydro," referring to water, and "philic," meaning loving or attracting. A substance that is hydrophilic may also be referred to, in a negative sense, as lipophobic. "Phobic" means fearing or hating, and thus lipophobic means lipid-hating, which therefore suggests that the chemical is water-loving.

If an organic molecule dissolves fully or partially in a nonaqueous or lipid solvent, the molecule is said to be lipophilic or to have lipophilic character. The term "lipophilic" or "lipid-loving" is synonymous with hydrophobic or water-hating, and these terms may be used interchangeably.

Hydrophilic	water-loving
Lipophobic	lipid-hating
Lipophilic	lipid-loving
Hydrophobic	water-hating

To predict whether a chemical will dissolve in water or a lipid solvent, it must be determined whether the molecule and its functional groups can bond to water or the lipid solvent molecules. THIS IS THE KEY TO SOLUBILITY. If a molecule, through its functional groups, can bond to water, it will show some degree of water solubility. If, on the other hand, a molecule cannot bond to water, but instead bonds to the molecules of a lipid solvent, it will be water-insoluble or lipid-soluble. Our goal is therefore to determine to what extent a molecule can or cannot bond to water. To do this, we must define the types of intermolecular bonding that can occur between molecules.

What are the types of intermolecular bonds?

VAN DER WAALS ATTRACTION (FORCES)

The weakest type of interaction is electrostatic in nature and is known as van der Waals attraction or van der Waals forces. This type of attraction occurs between the

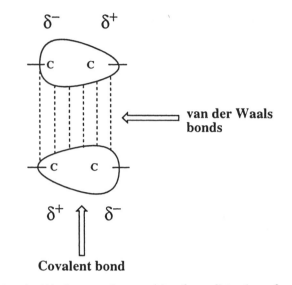

Covalent bond

FIGURE 1-1. Van der Waals attraction resulting from distortion of covalent bonds.

nonpolar portion of two molecules and is brought about by a mutual distortion of electron clouds making up the covalent bonds (Fig. 1-1). This attraction is also referred to as the induced dipole-induced dipole attraction. In addition to being weak, it is temperature-dependent, being important at low temperatures and of little significance at high temperatures. The attraction occurs only over a short distance, thus requiring a tight packing of molecules. Steric factors, such as molecular branching, strongly influence van der Waals attraction. This type of chemical force is most prevalent in hydrocarbon and aromatic systems. Van der Waals forces are approximately 0.5 to 1.0 kcal/mole for each atom involved. Van der Waals bonds are found in lipophilic solvents but are of little importance in water.

DIPOLE-DIPOLE BONDING (HYDROGEN BOND)

A stronger and important form of chemical bonding is the dipole-dipole bond, a specific example of which is the hydrogen bond (Fig. 1-2). A dipole results from the unequal sharing of a pair of electrons making up a covalent bond. This occurs

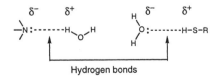

Hydrogen bonds

FIGURE 1-2. Hydrogen bonding of an amine to water and a thiol to water.

when the two atoms making up the covalent bond differ significantly in electronegativity. A partial ionic character develops in this portion of the molecule, leading to a permanent dipole, with the compound being described as a polar compound. The dipole-dipole attraction between two polar molecules arises from the negative end of one dipole being electrostatically attracted to the positive end of the second dipole. The hydrogen bond can occur when at least one dipole contains an electropositive hydrogen (e.g., a hydrogen covalently bonded to an electronegative atom such as oxygen, sulfur, nitrogen, or selenium), which in turn is attracted to a region of high electron density. Atoms with high electron densities are those with unshared pairs of electrons such as amine nitrogens, ether or alcohol oxygens, and thioether or thiol sulfurs. While hydrogen bonding is an example of dipole-dipole bonding, not all dipole-dipole bonding is hydrogen bonding (Fig. 1-3).

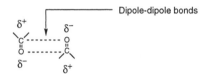

FIGURE 1-3. Dipole-dipole bonding between two ketone molecules.

Water, the important pharmaceutical solvent, is a good example of an hydrogen-bonding solvent. The ability of water to hydrogen bond accounts for the unexpectedly high boiling point of water as well as the characteristic dissolving properties of water. The hydrogen bond depends on temperature and distance. The energy of hydrogen bonding is 1.0 to 10.0 kcal/mole for each interaction.

IONIC ATTRACTION

A third type of bonding is the ionic attraction found quite commonly in inorganic molecules and salts of organic molecules. Ionic bonding results from the attraction of a negative atom for a positive atom (Fig. 1-4). The ionic bond involves a somewhat stronger attractive force of 5 kcal/mole or more and is least affected by temperature and distance.

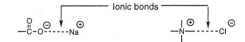

FIGURE 1-4. Ionic bonding found in salts of organic compounds.

ION-DIPOLE BONDING

Probably one of the most important chemical bonds involved in organic salts dissolving in water is the ion-dipole bond (Fig. 1-5). This bond occurs between an ion,

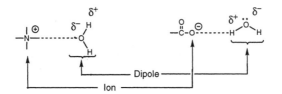

FIGURE 1-5. Ion-dipole bonding of a cationic amine to water and anionic carboxylic acid to water.

either cation or anion, and a formal dipole, such as is found in water. The following two types of interactions may exist:

1. A cation will show bonding to a region of high electron density in a dipole (e.g., the oxygen atom in water).
2. An anion will bond to an electron-deficient region in a dipole (e.g., the hydrogen atom in water).

Ion-dipole bonding is a strong attraction that is relatively insensitive to temperature or distance. When an organic compound with basic properties (e.g., an amine) is added to an aqueous acidic medium (pH below 7.0), the compound may form an ionic salt that, if dissociable, will have enhanced water solubility owing to ion-dipole bonding. Likewise, when an organic compound with acidic properties (e.g., carboxylic acids, phenols, unsubstituted or monosubstituted sulfonamides and unsubstituted imides) is added to an aqueous basic medium (pH above 7.0), the compound may form an ionic salt that, if dissociable, will have enhanced water solubility owing to ion-dipole bonding. Both of these examples are shown in Figure 1-5.

Water is an important solvent from both a pharmaceutical and a biologic standpoint. Therefore, when looking at any drug from a structural viewpoint, it is important to know whether the drug will dissolve in water. To predict water solubility, one must weigh the number and strength of hydrophilic groups in a molecule against the lipophilic groups present. If a molecule has a large amount of water-loving character, by interacting with water through hydrogen bonding or ion-dipole attraction, it would be expected to dissolve in water. If a molecule is deficient in hydrophilic groups but instead has a lipophilic portion capable of van der Waals attraction, then the molecule will most likely dissolve in a nonaqueous or lipophilic medium.

In reviewing the functional groups in organic chemistry, an attempt will be made to identify the lipophilic or hydrophilic character of each functional group.

Knowing the character of each functional group in a drug will then allow an intelligent prediction of the overall solubility of the molecule by weighing the importance of each type of interaction. This book is organized in such a way that each functional group is discussed individually. Yet, when dealing with a drug molecule, the student will usually find a polyfunctional molecule. The ultimate goal is that the student should be able to predict the solubility of actual drugs in water, aqueous acidic media, and aqueous basic media. Therefore, to use this book correctly and to prepare yourself for the typical complex drug molecules, it is recommended that you read through Chapter 18 after studying each functional group. This will help you put each functional group into perspective with respect to polyfunctional molecules.

Alkanes (C_nH_{2n+2})

■ **NOMENCLATURE.** The nomenclature of the alkanes may be either common or official nomenclature. The common nomenclature begins with the simplest system, methane, and proceeds to ethane, propane, butane, and so forth (Fig. 2-1). The "-ane" suffix indicates that the molecule is an alkane. This nomenclature works quite well until isomeric forms of the molecule appear (e.g., molecules with the same empirical formulas but different structural formulas). In butane, there are only two ways to put the molecule together, but as we consider larger molecules, many isomers are possible, and the nomenclature becomes unwieldy. Thus, a more systematic form of nomenclature is necessary. The IUPAC (International Union of Pure and Applied Chemistry) nomenclature is the official nomenclature.

IUPAC nomenclature requires that one find the longest continuous alkane chain. The name of this alkane chain becomes the base name. The chain is then numbered so as to provide the lowest possible numbers to the substituents. The number followed by the name of each substituent then precedes the base name of the straight-chain alkane. An example of naming an alkane according to IUPAC nomenclature is shown in Figure 2-2. The longest continuous chain is eight carbons.

This chain can be numbered from either end. Numbering left to right results in substituents at positions 2 (methyl), 5 (ethyl), and 7 (methyl). The name of this compound would be 5-ethyl-2,7-dimethyloctane. Numbering from right to left gives alkane substituents at the 2, 4, and 7 positions. This compound would be 4-ethyl-2,7-dimethyloctane. To determine which way to number, add the numbers that correspond to the substituent locations and choose the direction that gives the lowest sum. From left to right, one has 2 + 5 + 7, which equals 14. When num-

Structure	Common name
CH_4	Methane
CH_3-CH_3	Ethane
$CH_3-CH_2-CH_3$	Propane
$CH_3-CH_2-CH_2-CH_3$	*n*-Butane
$CH_3-\underset{\underset{CH_3}{\mid}}{CH}-CH_3$	*iso*-Butane

FIGURE 2-1. Common alkane nomenclature

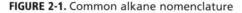

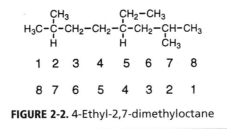

FIGURE 2-2. 4-Ethyl-2,7-dimethyloctane

bering from right to left, one has $2 + 4 + 7$, which equals 13. Therefore, the correct numbering system is from right to left, giving 4-ethyl-2,7-dimethyloctane. It should be noted that there is a convention for ordering the names of the substituents. The substituents are arranged in alphabetical order and appear before the base name of the molecule. Thus, ethyl precedes methyl. The number of groups present, in this case two methyls ("dimethyl") is not considered in this alphabetical arrangement.

■ **PHYSICAL-CHEMICAL PROPERTIES.** We wish to consider the following questions: Are alkanes going to be water-soluble, and can water solubility or the lack of it be explained? The physical-chemical properties of alkanes are readily understandable from the previous discussion of chemical bonding. These compounds are unable to undergo hydrogen bonding, ionic bonding, or ion-dipole bonding. The only intermolecular bonding possible with these compounds is the weak van der Waals attraction. For the smaller molecules with one to four carbon atoms, this bonding is not strong enough to hold the molecules together at room temperature, with the result that the lower-member alkanes are gases. For the larger molecules with 5 to 20 carbon atoms, the induced dipole-induced dipole interactions can occur, and the energy required to break the increased amount of bonding is more than is available at room temperature. The result is that the 5- to 20-carbon atom alkanes are liquids. One can see from Table 2-1 that the boiling point increases consistently as more van der Waals bonding occurs.

Table 2-1. BOILING POINTS OF COMMON ALKANES

ALKANE	BOILING POINT (°C)
Propane	−42.0
n-Butane	−0.5
n-Pentane	36.1
n-Hexane	69.0
n-Heptane	98.4
n-Octane	126.0

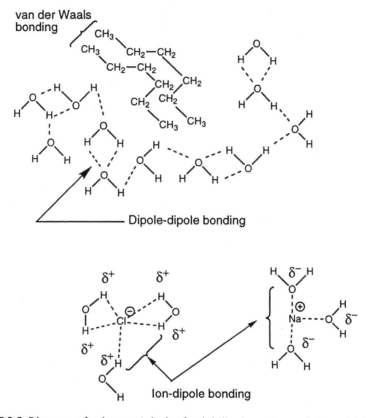

FIGURE 2-3. Diagram of *n*-hexane's lack of solubility in water and the solubility of sodium chloride in water through ion-dipole bonding.

The effects of adding an alkane to water are depicted in Figure 2-3. Water is an ordered medium with a considerable amount of inter-molecular bonding, indicated by its high boiling point (i.e., high in respect to its molecular weight). To dissolve in or to mix with water, foreign atoms must break into this lattice. Sodium chloride (table salt), which is quite water-soluble, is an example of a molecule capable of this. An alkane cannot break into the water lattice since it cannot bond to water. Ion-dipole interaction, which is possible for sodium chloride, is not possible for the alkane. Ionic bonding and hydrogen bonding between water and the alkane also are not possible. Van der Waals bonding between alkane and alkane is relatively strong, with little or no van der Waals attraction between the water and the alkane. The net result is that the alkane separates out and is immiscible in water. Alkanes will dissolve in a lipid solvent or oil layer. The term "lipid," "fat," or "oil," defined from the standpoint of solubility, means a water-immiscible or water-insoluble material. Lipid solvents are rich in alkane groups; therefore, it is not surprising that alkanes are soluble in lipid layers, since induced dipole-induced dipole bonding will be abundant. If an alkane has a choice between remaining in an aqueous area or moving to a lipid area, it will move to the lipid area. In chemistry, this means that if *n*-heptane is placed in a separatory funnel containing water and decane, the *n*-heptane will partition into the decane. This movement of alkanes also occurs in biologic systems and is best represented by the general anesthetic alkanes and their rapid partitioning into the lipid portion of the brain, while at the same time they have poor affinity for the aqueous blood. This concept will be discussed in detail in courses in medicinal chemistry.

Another property that should be mentioned is chemical stability. In the case of alkanes, one is dealing with a stable compound. For our purposes, these compounds are to be considered chemically inert to the conditions met "on the shelf"— namely, air, light, aqueous acid or base, and heat.

A final physical-chemical property that may be encountered in branched-chain alkanes is seen when a carbon atom is substituted with four different substituents (Fig. 2-4). Such a molecule is said to be asymmetric (that is, without a plane or point of symmetry) and is referred to as a chiral molecule. Chirality in a molecule means that the molecule exists as two stereoisomers, which are nonsuperimposable

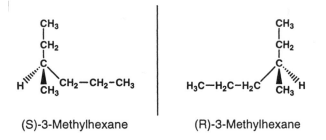

(S)-3-Methylhexane   (R)-3-Methylhexane

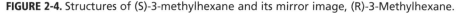

FIGURE 2-4. Structures of (S)-3-methylhexane and its mirror image, (R)-3-Methylhexane.

mirror images of each other, as shown in Figure 2-4. These stereoisomers are referred to as enantiomeric forms of the molecule and possess slightly different physical properties. In addition, chirality in a molecule usually leads to significant biological differences in biologically active molecules. The topic of stereoisomerism is reviewed briefly in Appendix A.

▪ **METABOLISM.** The alkane functional group is relatively nonreactive in vivo and will be excreted from the body unchanged. Although the student should consider the alkanes themselves as nonreactive and the alkane portions of a drug as nonreactive, several notable exceptions will be emphasized in the medicinal chemistry courses, and they should be learned as exceptions. Two such exceptions are shown

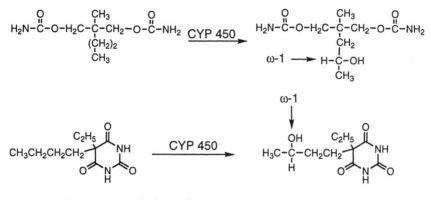

FIGURE 2-5. Metabolism of meprobamate and butylbarbital.

in Figure 2-5. When metabolism does occur, it is commonly an oxidation reaction catalyzed by a cytochrome P450 isoform (CYP 450) previously known as mixed-function oxidase enzymes, and in most cases it occurs at the end of the hydrocarbon, the omega carbon, or adjacent to the final carbon at the omega-minus-one carbon, as shown. For additional discussion of the metabolic process see Appendix C, Metabolism.

Alkenes (C_nH_{2n})

3

■ **NOMENCLATURE.** The common nomenclature for the alkenes uses the radical name representing the total number of carbons present and the suffix "-ene," which indicates the presence of a double bond (Fig. 3-1). This type of nomenclature becomes awkward for branched-chain alkenes, and the official IUPAC nomenclature becomes useful. With IUPAC nomenclature, the longest continuous chain containing the double bond is chosen and is given a base name that corresponds to the alkane of that length. As indicated in Figure 3-2, the longest chain has seven carbons and is therefore a heptane derivative. The chain is numbered so as to assign the lowest possible number to the double bond. In numbering left to right, the double bond is at the 3 position, which is preferred, rather than numbering right to left, which would put the double bond at the 4 position. With the molecule correctly numbered, the final step in naming the compound consists of naming and numbering the alkyl radicals, followed by the location of the double

Structure	Common name
$CH_2=CH_2$	Ethylene
$CH_2=CH-CH_3$	Propylene
$CH_2=CH-CH_2-CH_3$	1-Butylene
$CH_2=\underset{\underset{CH_3}{\mid}}{C}-CH_3$	*iso-* Butylene

FIGURE 3-1. Common alkene nomenclature.

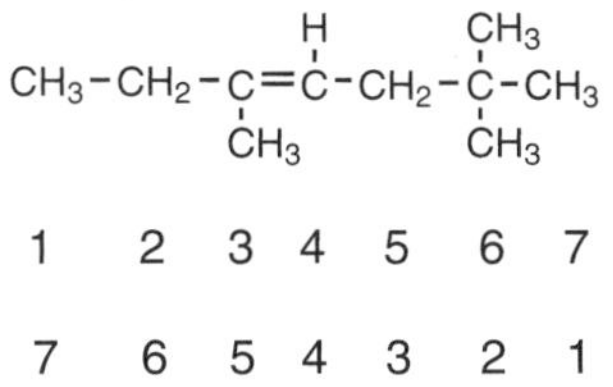

$$CH_3-CH_2-\underset{\underset{CH_3}{\mid}}{C}=\overset{\overset{H}{\mid}}{C}-CH_2-\underset{\underset{CH_3}{\mid}}{\overset{\overset{CH_3}{\mid}}{C}}-CH_3$$

| 1 | 2 | 3 | 4 | 5 | 6 | 7 |

| 7 | 6 | 5 | 4 | 3 | 2 | 1 |

FIGURE 3-2. 3,6,6-Trimethyl-3-heptene

bond and the alkane name, in which the "-ane" is dropped and replaced with the "-ene." In the example, the correct name would be 3,6,6-trimethyl-3 (the location of the double bond) hept (seven carbons) ene (meaning an alkene).

The introduction of a double bond into a molecule also raises the possibility of geometric isomers. Isomers are compounds with the same empirical formula but a different structural formula. If the difference in structural formulas comes from lack of free rotation around a bond, this is referred to as a geometric isomer. 2-Butene may exist as a *trans*-2-butene or *cis*-2-butene, which are examples of geometric isomers (Fig. 3-3). The "E,Z" nomenclature has been instituted to deal with tri- and tetra-substituted alkenes, which cannot be readily named by cis/trans nomenclature. The "E" is taken from the German word *entgegen*, which means opposite, and the "Z" from *zusammen*, meaning together. Using a series of priority rules, if the two substituents of highest priority are on the same side of the π bond, the configuration of Z is assigned, whereas if the two high-priority groups are on opposite sides, the E configuration is used. In the example in Figure 3-2, the correct nomenclature becomes (E)-3,6,6-trimethyl-3-heptene.

■ **PHYSICAL-CHEMICAL PROPERTIES.** The physical properties of the alkenes are similar to those of the alkanes. The lower members, having two through four carbon atoms, are gases at room temperature. Alkenes with five carbon atoms or more are liquids with increasing boiling points corresponding to increases in molecular weight. The weak intermolecular interaction that accounts for the low boiling point

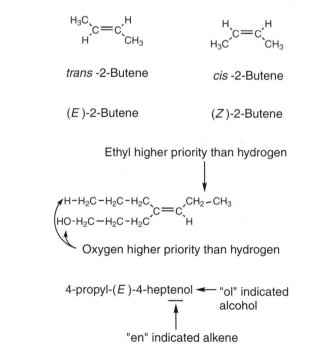

FIGURE 3-3. Examples of E,Z nomenclature for naming alkenes.

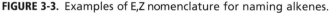

is again of the induced dipole-induced dipole type. Recognizing what type of inter-molecular interaction is possible also allows a prediction of nonaqueous versus aqueous solubility. Since alkenes cannot hydrogen bond and have a weak perma-nent dipole, they cannot dissolve in the aqueous layer. Alkenes will dissolve in non-polar solvents such as lipids, fats, or oil layers. Therefore, the physical properties of alkenes parallel those of the alkanes. When the chemical properties are considered, a departure from similarity to the alkane is found. The multiple bond gives the mol-ecule a reactive site. From a pharmaceutical standpoint, alkenes are prone to oxi-dation, leading to peroxide formation (Fig. 3-4). Peroxides are quite unstable and may explode. In addition, alkenes, especially the volatile members, are quite flam-mable and may explode in the presence of oxygen and a spark.

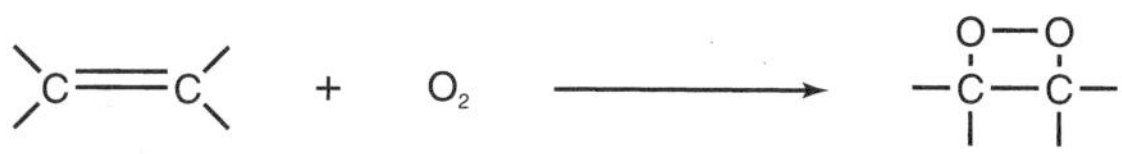

$$\text{C}=\text{C} \quad + \quad O_2 \quad \longrightarrow \quad -\overset{O-O}{\underset{|}{\text{C}}}-\overset{}{\underset{|}{\text{C}}}-$$

FIGURE 3-4. Oxidation of an alkene with molecular oxygen leading to a peroxide.

■ **METABOLISM.** Metabolism of the alkenes, as with the previously discussed alkanes, is not common. For our purposes, the alkene functional group should be considered metabolically stable. While alkene-containing drugs are usually stable in the body, the alkene functional groups of several body metabolites serve as cen-ters of reaction (Fig. 3-5). The unsaturated fatty acids add water to give alcohols. A

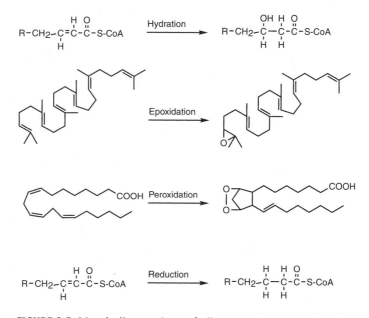

FIGURE 3-5. Metabolic reactions of alkene-containing molecules.

cytochrome P450 oxidase attacks the alkene functional group in squalene to give an epoxide during the biosynthesis of steroids. A peroxide intermediate is formed from eicosatrienoate, a triene, during prostaglandin biosynthesis, and during saturated fatty acid synthesis, alkenes are reduced in vivo. You should be familiar, therefore, with these possible reactions of the alkene functional group and should not be surprised if an alkene-containing drug is metabolized.

CYCLOALKANES: ALKENE ISOMERS

Before leaving the topic of alkenes, a group of compounds that are isomeric to the alkenes should be mentioned. The cycloalkanes have the same empirical formula, C_nH_{2n}, as the alkenes but possess a different structural formula and are therefore isomeric. Three important members of this class are cyclopropane, cyclopentane, and cyclohexane (Fig. 3-6). Cyclopropane acts chemically like propene, while cyclopentane and cyclohexane are chemically inert, much like the alkanes. All three compounds are lipid-soluble and quite flammable. The latter two ring systems are common to many drug molecules.

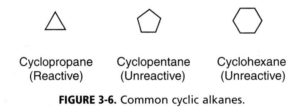

Cyclopropane   Cyclopentane   Cyclohexane
(Reactive)   (Unreactive)   (Unreactive)

FIGURE 3-6. Common cyclic alkanes.

Similar to the alkenes, the cycloalkanes do not show free rotation around the carbon-carbon bonds of the cycloalkane and as a result have the potential of geometric isomers. With polysubstituted cycloalkanes *cis* and *trans* isomers exist, resulting in compounds with different physical-chemical properties. An added characteristic of cycloalkanes with six or more carbons (less so with cyclopentane) is the ability of the molecule to exist in different conformational forms or isomers. While conformational isomers of a molecule (that is, the way the molecule stands in space) do not change the physical-chemical properties of a molecule, nor are these isomers separable, conformational isomers of a molecule may affect the way

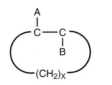

trans isomer

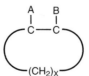

cis isomer

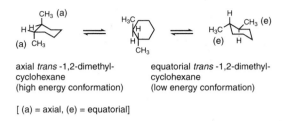

axial *trans* -1,2-dimethyl-
cyclohexane
(high energy conformation)

equatorial *trans* -1,2-dimethyl-
cyclohexane
(low energy conformation)

[(a) = axial, (e) = equatorial]

FIGURE 3-7. Examples of the conformational isomers of trans-1,2,-dimethylcyclohexane.

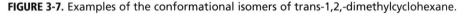

that the molecule is drawn. As an example, *trans* 1,2-dimethylcyclohexane has a high energy conformation drawn with the methyl groups in their axial conformation and a low energy conformation with the methyls in the equatorial conformation (Fig. 3-7). The significance of conformational isomers of a molecule becomes important when considering drug-receptor interactions and will be discussed in medicinal chemistry courses.

Aromatic Hydrocarbons

4

■ **NOMENCLATURE.** Another class of hydrocarbons, shown in Figure 4-1, is the aromatic hydrocarbons. In aromatic nomenclature, a single name is used for the aromatic nucleus. Several of the most common nuclei have been shown, along with their official name and numbering system.

■ **PHYSICAL-CHEMICAL PROPERTIES.** At first glance, it might be thought that the aromatic hydrocarbons are nothing more than cyclic alkenes, but this is not the case. Remember that aromatic compounds do not have isolated single and double bonds; instead, they have a cloud of electrons above and below the ring. This is a cloud of delocalized electrons that are not as readily available as the electrons in the alkenes. The aromatic systems are therefore not as prone to the chemical reactions that affect alkenes.

Formation of peroxides, a potentially serious pharmaceutical problem with many alkenes, is not considered a problem with the aromatic hydrocarbons. The typical reaction of the aromatic systems is the electrophilic reaction. In the electrophilic reaction, the electrophile, the electron-loving, positively charged species, attacks the electron-dense cloud of the aromatic ring. There is one significant elec-

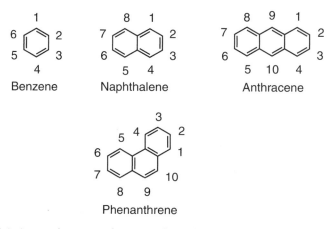

FIGURE 4-1. Aromatic nomenclature and numbering of common aromatic rings.

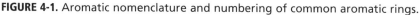

trophilic reaction that occurs only in biologic systems, and this is known as hydroxylation. This reaction is quite important during drug metabolism but does not occur in vitro. Aromatic hydrocarbons are quite stable on the shelf. These hydrocarbons, like other hydrocarbons, are lipophilic and flammable. Because of their high electron density and flat nature, however, aromatic hydrocarbons show a somewhat stronger capacity to bond through van der Waals attraction. Aromatic rings appear to play a significant role in the binding of a drug to biologic proteins, as will be seen in courses on medicinal chemistry.

■ **METABOLISM.** As already mentioned, aromatic rings are quite prone to oxidation in vivo or, more specifically, to aromatic hydroxylation. This reaction commonly occurs with several of the cytochrome P450 isoforms and may involve an initial epoxidation. In a few cases, this highly reactive epoxide has been isolated, but in most cases the epoxide rearranges to give the hydroxylation product, the phenol or dialcohol, as shown in Figure 4-2. The importance of this reaction is considerable.

Aromatic hydroxylation significantly increases the water solubility of the aromatic system (See Chapter 7, Phenols). In many cases this results in a rapid removal of the chemical from the body, while in a few cases hydroxylation may actually increase the activity of the drug. An area of considerable importance has been the study of the role of hydroxylation of aromatic hydrocarbons and its relationship to the carcinogenic properties of aromatic hydrocarbons. Evidence suggests that the intermediate epoxides are responsible for this carcinogenic effect.

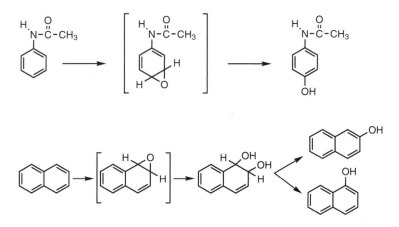

FIGURE 4-2. Aromatic hydroxylation catalyzed by Cytochrome P450 (CYP 450).

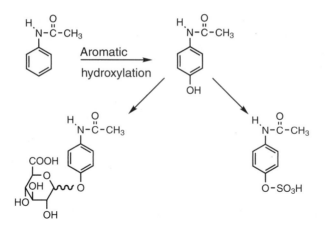

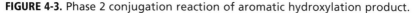

FIGURE 4-3. Phase 2 conjugation reaction of aromatic hydroxylation product.

As indicated, the phenols formed by aromatic hydroxylation may be eliminated as such from the body or may undergo a phase 2 conjugation, giving rise to a sulfate conjugate or a glucuronide conjugate, as shown in Figure 4-3. These conjugates exhibit an even greater water solubility (see Appendix C, Metabolism for discussion of conjugation reactions).

Halogenated Hydrocarbons

■ **NOMENCLATURE.** The common nomenclature for mono-substituted halogenated hydrocarbons consists of the name of the alkyl radical followed by the name of the halogen atom. Examples of this nomenclature, along with the structures and names of several common polyhalogenated hydrocarbons, are shown in Figure 5-1.

This nomenclature again becomes complicated as the branching of the hydrocarbon chain increases, and one therefore uses IUPAC nomenclature. The IUPAC nomenclature requires choosing the longest continuous hydrocarbon chain, followed by numbering of the chain so as to assign the lowest number to the halide. The compound is then named as a haloalkane. This is illustrated in Figure 5-2 for 2-bromo-4-methylpentane.

Structure	Common name
$CH_3 \cdot F$	Methylfluoride
$CH_3 - CH_2 - Cl$	Ethylchloride
$CH_3 - CH_2 - CH_2 \, Br$	Propylbromide
$CH_3 - CH_2 - CH_2 - CH_2 - I$	*n*-Butyliodide
CH_2Cl_2	Methylene chloride
$CHCl_3$	Chloroform
CCl_4	Carbon tetrachloride
$Cl - CH_2 - CH_2 - Cl$	Ethylene chloride

FIGURE 5-1. Common halogenated hydrocarbon nomenclature.

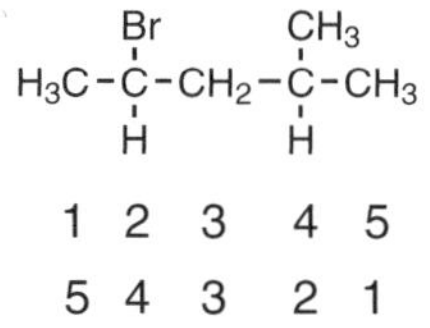

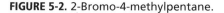

$$\begin{array}{ccc} Br & & CH_3 \\ | & & | \\ H_3C - C - CH_2 - C - CH_3 \\ | & & | \\ H & & H \end{array}$$

$$\begin{array}{ccccc} 1 & 2 & 3 & 4 & 5 \\ 5 & 4 & 3 & 2 & 1 \end{array}$$

FIGURE 5-2. 2-Bromo-4-methylpentane.

■ **PHYSICAL-CHEMICAL PROPERTIES.** The properties of the halogenated hydrocarbons are different from those of the hydrocarbons previously discussed. The monohaloalkanes have a permanent dipole owing to the strongly electronegative halide attached to the carbon. The permanent dipole does not guarantee dipole-dipole bonding, however. Although the halogen is rich in electron density, there is no region highly deficient in electrons, and intermolecular bonding is therefore weak and again depends on the van der Waals attraction. Since only van der Waals bonding is possible, these compounds have low boiling points and poor water solubility. The halogens covalently bound to carbon in general increase the lipophilic nature of the compounds to which they are bound. Another property of the halogenated hydrocarbons is a decrease in flammability with an increase in the number of halogens. In fact, carbon tetrachloride has been used in fire extinguishers. In general, these compounds are highly lipid-soluble and chemically nonreactive.

One important chemical reaction that methylene chloride, chloroform, and several other polyhalogenated compounds undergo is shown in Figure 5-3. Chloroform, in the presence of oxygen and heat, is converted to phosgene, a reactive and toxic chemical. To destroy any phosgene that may form in a bottle of chloroform, a small amount of alcohol is usually present. The alcohol reacts with the phosgene to give a nontoxic carbonate.

■ **METABOLISM.** The lack of chemical reactivity in vitro carries over to in vivo stability. In general, halogenated hydrocarbons are not readily metabolized. This stability significantly increases the potential for human toxicity. Since the compounds are quite lipid-soluble, they are not readily excreted by the kidney. Since they are not rapidly metabolized to water-soluble agents, the halogenated hydrocarbons tend to have a prolonged biologic half-life, increasing the likelihood for systemic toxicity. This may also account for the potential carcinogenic properties of some halogenated hydrocarbons.

In summary, one significant property is common to all of the hydrocarbons, and that is the lack of ability to bond to water and thus the lipophilic or hydrophobic nature. SINCE ALL ORGANIC MOLECULES HAVE A HYDROCARBON PORTION, THIS PROPERTY WILL SHOW UP TO SOME EXTENT IN ALL MOLECULES. You will have to weigh the extent of influence of the lipophilic portion against the quantity of hydrophilic character to predict whether a molecule will dissolve in a nonaqueous medium or in water.

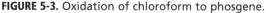

FIGURE 5-3. Oxidation of chloroform to phosgene.

Alcohols

■ **NOMENCLATURE.** The common nomenclature of alcohols is to name the molecule as an "alcohol" preceded by the names of the hydrocarbon radical (Fig. 6-1). Methyl and ethyl alcohol are examples of primary alcohols, isopropyl alcohol is an example of a secondary alcohol, and tertiary butyl alcohol is an example of a tertiary alcohol. The primary, secondary, and tertiary designations given to an alcohol depend upon the number of carbons that are attached to the carbon that contains the OH group. The primary designation indicates that one carbon is attached to the carbon bearing the OH group; the secondary designation indicates that two carbons are attached; and the tertiary designation indicates that three carbons are attached.

Once again, the nomenclature becomes clumsy as the hydrocarbon portion branches, and the official IUPAC nomenclature must be used (see Fig. 6-1). The longest continuous chain that contains the hydroxyl group is chosen. The chain is then numbered to give the lowest number to the hydroxyl group. Other substituents, preceded by their numbered location, come first, followed by the location of the hydroxyl group, followed by the name of the alkane. To show that this is an alcohol, the "e" is dropped from the alkane name and replaced by "ol," the official sign of an alcohol.

■ **PHYSICAL-CHEMICAL PROPERTIES.** The properties of the alcohol offer a departure from the compounds that have been discussed previously. The OH group can

Structure	Common name	IUPAC name
$CH_3·OH$	Methyl alcohol (Wood alcohol)	Methanol
CH_3-CH_2-OH	Ethyl alcohol (Alcohol USP)	Ethanol
$CH_3-CH-OH$ $\quad CH_3$	Isopropyl alcohol (Rubbing alcohol)	2-Propanol
$\quad CH_3$ CH_3-C-OH $\quad CH_3$	*tert*-Butyl alcohol	2-Methyl-2-propanol

FIGURE 6-1. Common and IUPAC nomenclature for alcohols.

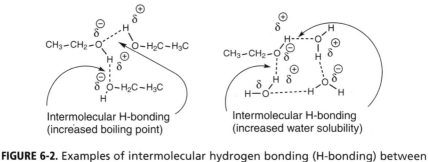

Intermolecular H-bonding (increased boiling point)

Intermolecular H-bonding (increased water solubility)

FIGURE 6-2. Examples of intermolecular hydrogen bonding (H-bonding) between molecules of ethanol and between ethanol and water.

participate in intermolecular hydrogen bonding (Fig. 6-2). Because of the electronegativity of the oxygen and the electropositive proton, a permanent dipole exists. The hydrogen attached to the oxygen is slightly positive in nature and the oxygen slightly negative. Remember, this is not a formal charge but simply an unequal sharing of the pair of electrons that make up the covalent bond. The intermolecular hydrogen bonding that is now possible between the alcohol molecules results in relatively high boiling points compared with their hydrocarbon counterparts (Table 6-1). Also important is the fact that the alcohol group can hydrogen bond to water (see Fig. 6-2). This means that it can break into the water lattice, with the result that the alcohol functional group promotes water solubility. The extent of water solubility for each alcohol will depend on the size of the hydrocarbon portion (see Table 6-1). C_1 through C_3 alcohols are miscible with water in all proportions. As the length of the hydrocarbon chain increases, the hydrophilic nature of the molecule decreases. The location of the hydroxyl radical also influences water solubility, although not as dramatically as chain length. A hydroxyl group centered in the molecule will have a greater potential

TABLE 6-1. BOILING POINTS AND WATER SOLUBILITY OF COMMON ALCOHOLS

	Boiling Points °C	Solubility (g/100g H_2O)
Methanol	65.5	∞
Ethanol	78.3	∞
1-Propanol	97.0	∞
2-Propanol	82.4	∞
1-Butanol	117.2	7.9
2-Butanol	99.5	12.5
1-Pentanol	137.3	2.3

for producing water solubility than a hydroxyl at the end of the straight chain. If a second hydroxyl is added, solubility is increased. An example of this is 1,5-pentanediol. It can be thought of as ethanol and propanol put together. Since both alcohols are quite water-soluble, it would be predicted that 1,5-pentanediol would also be quite water-soluble, and it is. It also follows that as the solubility of the alcohol in water decreases, the solubility of the alcohol in nonaqueous media increases. In summary, it can be said that an alcohol functional group has the ability to solubilize to the extent of 1% or greater an alkane chain of five or six carbon atoms.

Looking at the chemical reactivity of the alcohol, we find that from a pharmaceutical standpoint the alcohol functional group is a relatively stable unit. Remember, though, that in the presence of oxidizing agents, a primary alcohol will be oxidized to a carboxylic acid after passing through an intermediate aldehyde (Fig. 6-3). The secondary alcohols can be oxidized to a ketone, and a tertiary alcohol is stable to mild oxidation. The oxidation of an alcohol in vitro is not commonly encountered because of the limited number of oxidating agents used pharmaceutically.

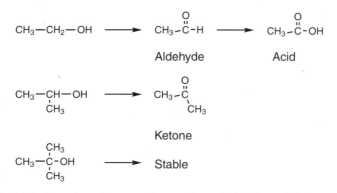

FIGURE 6-3. Oxidation of a primary and secondary alcohol by oxidizing agents (normally uncommon in pharmaceutical products).

■ **METABOLISM.** Although the alcohol functional group is relatively stable in vitro, it is readily metabolized in the body by a variety of enzymes, most notably cytochrome P450 enzymes and alcohol dehydrogenase. Both primary and secondary alcohols are prone to oxidation by oxidase enzymes, resulting in the formation of carboxylic acids or ketones, respectively (Fig. 6-4). The tertiary alcohols are stable to oxidase enzymes. Another common metabolic fate of the alcohol is conjugation with glucuronic acid to give a glucuronide or with sulfuric acid to give the sulfate conjugate. Both of these conjugates show a considerable increase in water solubility. The glucuronide has several additional alcohol functional groups that exhib-

Oxidation:

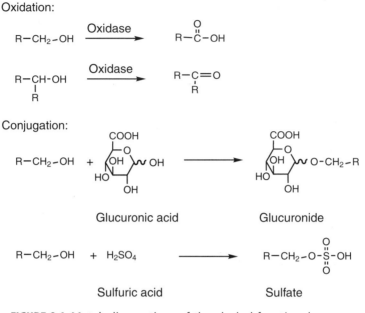

Conjugation:

FIGURE 6-4. Metabolic reactions of the alcohol functional group.

it dipole-dipole bonding to water. The alcohol is conjugated to the glucuronic acid as an acetal through an "ether-like" linkage, while the conjugation to sulfuric acid is as an ester linkage.

When the alcohol combines with sulfuric acid, it is excreted as a sulfate conjugate, which would also be expected to show considerable water solubility because of the hydrogen bonding and ion-dipole bonding afforded by the sulfate portion of the molecule. These latter reactions are considered phase 2 metabolisms (see Appendix C, Metabolism).

Phenols

■ **NOMENCLATURE.** Phenols may appear to have some similarity to the alcohol functional group, but they are considerably different in several aspects. Phenols differ from alcohols by having the OH group attached directly to an aromatic ring. The nomenclature of the phenols is not as systematic as has been the case with the previous functional groups. In many cases, phenols are named as substituted phenols using the common ortho, meta, or para nomenclature for the location of the substituents, or the official nomenclature, in which the ring is numbered, with the carbon that bears the OH being assigned the 1 position (Fig. 7-1). In phenol nomenclature, common names are often used, such as cresol, catechol, and resorcinol. Therefore, one must be aware of these common names as well as the official nomenclature.

■ **PHYSICAL-CHEMICAL PROPERTIES.** In considering the physical properties of the phenols, one is again aware of the OH group, in which a strong electronegative group, oxygen, is attached to the electropositive hydrogen. The permanent dipole is capable of intermolecular hydrogen bonding, which results in high boiling points

Structure	Common name	IUPAC name
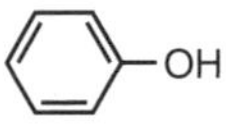 ⬡—OH	Carbolic acid	Phenol
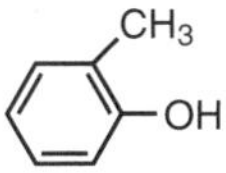 ⬡(CH₃)—OH	o-Cresol	2-Methylphenol
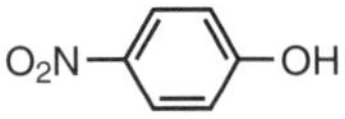 O₂N—⬡—OH	p-Nitrophenol	4-Nitrophenol
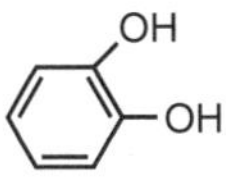 ⬡(OH)—OH	Catechol	1,2-Dihydroxybenzene
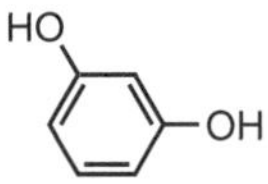 HO—⬡—OH	Resorcinol	1,3-Dihydroxybenzene
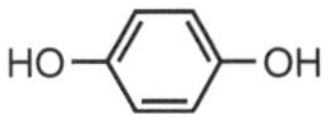 HO—⬡—OH	Hydroquinone	1,4-Dihydroxybenzene

FIGURE 7-1. Phenol nomenclature.

Table 7-1. BOILING POINTS AND WATER SOLUBILITY OF COMMON PHENOLS

	BOILING POINT °C	SOLUBILITY (g/100g H_2O)
Cyclohexanol	161	3.6
Phenol	182	9.3
p-Cresol	202	2.3
m-Chlorophenol	214	2.6
Catechol	246	45.0

and water solubility. Added to the list of compounds in Table 7-1 is cyclohexanol. Cyclohexanol differs from phenol only in the lack of the aromatic ring. The change in the boiling point and solubility in going from cyclohexanol to phenol may seem rather large, and indeed it should be, since one property becomes important with phenols that is absent in alcohols: that property is *acidity*.

Before discussing the acidity of the phenols, let us look at some additional factors that affect solubility. As the lipophilic nature of the phenol is increased, the water solubility is decreased. The addition of a methyl (cresol) or a halogen (chlorophenol) greatly reduces the water solubility of these compounds (see Table 7-1). The addition of a second hydroxyl, such as in catechol, increases water solubility, as was the case with the previous diols. The solubility of catechol will again greatly decrease as alkyls are added to this molecule.

The acidity of phenol and substituted phenols is considered in the following illustration (Fig. 7-2). First, an acid must be defined. The classic definition states that an acid is a chemical that has the ability to give up a proton. Phenol has this ability and can therefore be considered an acid. The ease with which this proton is given up (dissociation) will influence the ratio of K_1 to K_{-1} (see Fig. 7-2). If K_1 is much greater than K_{-1}, a strong acid exists, while if K_1 is smaller than K_{-1}, a weak acid results. The factor that influences the ratio of K_1 to K_{-1} is the stability of the anion formed (in this case the phenolate anion). It should be recalled that the phenolate anion can be stabilized by resonance (that is, the overlap of the pair of electrons on the oxygen with the delocalized cloud of electrons above and below the aromatic ring; see Fig. 7-2). This is something an alcohol cannot do because an alcohol hydroxyl is not adjacent to an aromatic system, and resonance stabilization does not occur. Therefore, dissociation of the hydrogen from the oxygen is not possible in alcohols and, by definition, the inability to give up a proton means that the alcohol is not acidic but neutral.

Let us return now to the question of boiling points and solubilities of alcohols versus phenols. Alcohols as neutral polar groups are only capable of participating in a hydrogen-bonding interaction with water. On the other hand, phenols, due to their acidity, exist both as neutral molecules and (to some extent) as ions; therefore,

Acid (definition): HX + H_2O $\underset{K_{-1}}{\overset{K_1}{\rightleftharpoons}}$ $H_3O^{\oplus}$ + $X^{\ominus}$

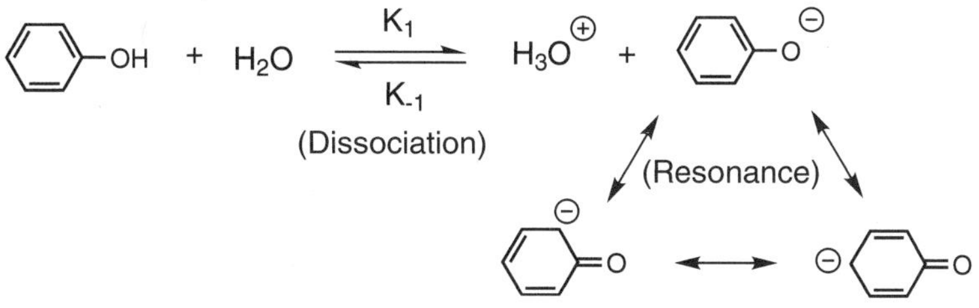

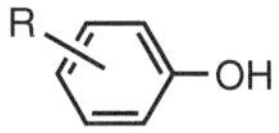

$C_6H_5{-}OH$ + H_2O $\underset{K_{-1}}{\overset{K_1}{\rightleftharpoons}}$ $H_3O^{\oplus}$ + $C_6H_5{-}O^{\ominus}$

(Dissociation)

(Resonance)

$R{-}C_6H_4{-}OH$	Dissociation Constant	
	Ka (in water)	pKa
R = H	1.1×10^{-10}	9.96
R = m-CH$_3$	9.8×10^{-11}	10.01
R = p-CH$_3$	6.7×10^{-11}	10.17
R = m-NO$_2$	5.0×10^{-9}	8.3
R = p-NO$_2$	6.9×10^{-8}	7.16
Mineral acids	10^{-1}	1.0
Carboxylic acids	10^{-5}	5.0
Alcohols	10^{-17}	17.0

FIGURE 7-2. Dissociation constants and pKa's in water for common phenols.

not only will hydrogen bonding occur, but also the stronger ion-dipole bonding can occur between the phenol and water. The prediction of a higher boiling point and a greater water solubility relates to the presence of ion-dipole interaction as well as dipole-dipole bonding.

The acidity of phenols is influenced by the substitution on the aromatic ring. Substitution ortho to the phenol affects acidity in an unpredictable manner, while substitution meta or para to the phenol results in acidities that are predictable. Substitution with a group capable of donating electrons into the aromatic ring decreases acidity. The most pronounced effect occurs when the substitution is para or in direct conjugation. Addition of an electron-withdrawing group to the aromatic ring results in increased acidity. Again, the most pronounced effect occurs with para substitution. In both cases, the influence of substituents on acidity comes from the inability or ability of the substituent to stabilize the phenolate form.

Comparison of the acidity of phenols to that of carboxylic acids and mineral acids demonstrates that phenols are weak acids.

Another significant property of phenols is their chemical reactivity. An important reaction is shown in Figure 7-3. Because phenol is a weak acid, it will not react with sodium bicarbonate, a weak base, but will react with strong bases such as sodium hydroxide or potassium hydroxide to give the respective phenolate salts. Salt

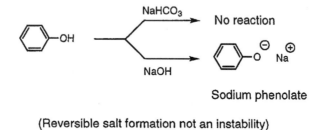

Sodium phenolate

(Reversible salt formation not an instability)

FIGURE 7-3. Acid-base reaction between phenol and a strong base.

formation is an important reaction since the phenolates formed are ions and will dissolve in water through the much stronger ion-dipole bonding. As salts, the simple phenols (phenol, cresol, and chlorophenol) are extremely soluble in water. Several words of caution are necessary before leaving this topic. Sodium and potassium salts will greatly increase the water solubility of the phenols. Heavy metal salts of the phenols will actually become less water-soluble because of the inability of the salt to dissociate in water. Salts of phenols that are capable of dissociation in water will always increase water solubility, and for most of the phenols of medicinal value, the salts will give enough solubility so that the drug will dissolve in water at the concentration needed for biologic activity. As the lipophilic portions attached to the aromatic ring increase, however, the solubility of the phenolate salts will decrease. *You should realize that while salt formation* (with a dissociating salt) *is an example of a chemical reaction, it is not a chemical instability.* Treatment of the water-soluble salt with acid will reverse this reaction, regenerating the phenol. For our purposes, salt formation resulting in precipitation of the organic molecule is a pharmaceutical incompatibility that the student should watch for.

A second significant chemical reaction of phenols involves their facile air oxidation. Phenols are oxidized to quinones, which are highly colored. A clear solution of phenol allowed to stand in contact with air or light soon develops a yellow coloration owing to the formation of *p*-quinone or *o*-quinone (Fig. 7-4). This reaction occurs more readily with salts of phenols and with polyphenolic compounds. Phenols and their salts must be protected from oxygen and light by being stored in closed, amber containers or by the addition of antioxidants.

■ **METABOLISM.** The metabolism of phenols is much like that of alcohols. The

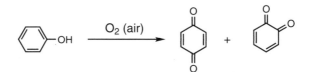

FIGURE 7-4. Oxidation of phenol with molecular oxygen.

phenol may be oxidized, or, using the terminology previously used for aromatic oxidation, the phenol may be hydroxylated, to give a diphenolic compound (Fig. 7-5) (phase 1 reaction). In most cases, the new OH group will be either ortho or para to the original hydroxyl group. Hydroxylation reactions are commonly catalyzed by members of the cytochrome P450 family of enzymes. The most common form of metabolism of phenols is conjugation with glucuronic acid to form the glucuronide or sulfonation to give the sulfate conjugate (phase 2 reaction). Both conjugation reactions give metabolites that have greater water solubility than the unmetabolized phenol. An additional type of metabolism seen to a minor extent is methylation of the phenol to give the methyl ether. This type of reaction will actually decrease water solubility.

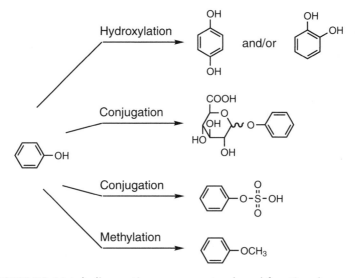

FIGURE 7-5. Metabolic reactions common to phenol functional groups.

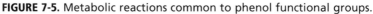

Ethers

■ **NOMENCLATURE.** Another important functional group found in many medicinal agents is the ether moiety shown in Figure 8-1. The ethers use a common nomenclature in which the compounds are called ethers, and both substituents are named by their radical names, such as methyl, ethyl, or phenyl. Thus, Ether USP, a common name, can also be referred to as diethylether. The official names for the simple ethers are shown in Figure 8-1. The inherent problem of naming the alkyl radical again arises as branching in the alkyl chain occurs. The official nomenclature names the compounds as alkoxy derivatives of alkanes. In the example shown below, the longest continuous alkane chain containing the ether is chosen as the base name, and the alkane is numbered to give the ether the lowest number. The correct name for the ether is therefore 2-methoxy (numbered to give the alkoxy the lowest number)-4,4-dimethylpentane (the longest alkane chain).

■ **PHYSICAL-CHEMICAL PROPERTIES.** What can one predict about the water solubility of the ether group? It is interesting that the synthesis of ethers is brought about by combining two alcohols or an alcohol and phenol to give the ether. The precursors have high boiling points, strongly bond to water to give solubility, and show chemical reactivity under certain conditions. Ethers, by contrast, are low-boiling liquids with poor water solubility (Fig. 8-2) and chemically are almost inert.

Structure	Common name (Alkylalkylether)	IUPAC name
$H_3C-O-CH_2CH_3$	Ethylmethylether	Methoxyethane
$CH_3CH_2-O-CH_2CH_3$	Diethylether (Ether U.S.P.)	Ethoxyethane
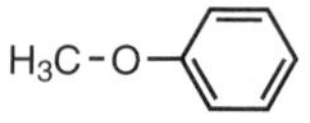 $H_3C-O-\langle\ \rangle$	Methylphenylether (Anisole)	Methoxybenzene

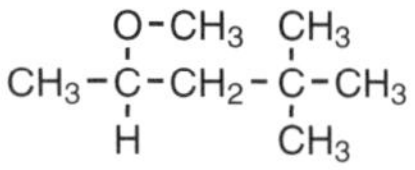

$$
\begin{array}{ccccc}
& O-CH_3 & & CH_3 & \\
CH_3-&C-CH_2-&&C-CH_3 & \\
& H & & CH_3 &
\end{array}
$$

1	2	3	4	5	2-Methoxy-4,4-dimethylpentane (Correct)
5	4	3	2	1	4-Methoxy-2,2-dimethylpentane (Incorrect)

FIGURE 8-1. Ether nomenclature.

Dipole-dipole bond (H-bond)

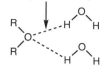

Ether

Ether	Solubility (g/100 ml H_2O)
R = C_2H_5	8.4
R = 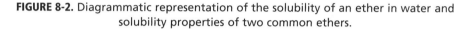	0.002

FIGURE 8-2. Diagrammatic representation of the solubility of an ether in water and solubility properties of two common ethers.

This becomes understandable when one recalls that the properties of alcohols and phenols depend primarily upon the OH group. With diethyl ether, resulting from the combination of two moles of ethanol, the OH groups have been lost. Without the OH group, hydrogen bonds cannot exist, and the only intermolecular bonding is weak van der Waals attraction and thus a low boiling point. Ether can hydrogen bond to water. The hydrogen of water will bond to the electron-rich oxygen (see Fig. 8-2). The lower-membered ethers therefore show partial water solubility, but as the hydrocarbon portion increases, water solubility rapidly decreases. In the area of general anesthetics, this water solubility for ethers has a significant effect on the onset and duration of biologic activity. The figures given for water solubility for two ethers shown in Figure 8-2 demonstrate how rapidly water solubility decreases as the hydrocarbon portion increases.

Chemically the ethers are relatively nonreactive, stable entities, with one important exception. Liquid ethers in contact with atmospheric oxygen form *peroxides* (Fig. 8-3). The peroxide formed, although not present in great quantities, can be quite irritating to the mucous membranes and, if concentrated, may explode. Hence, care should be taken in handling ethers to minimize the contact with oxygen. Many times an antioxidant such as copper metal is added to take up any oxygen that may be present and thus prevent this instability.

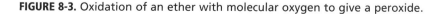

FIGURE 8-3. Oxidation of an ether with molecular oxygen to give a peroxide.

■ **METABOLISM.** The metabolism of ethers in general is uneventful. With most ethers, one finds the ether excreted unchanged. There are exceptions to this rule, and the one exception that should be learned is the metabolic dealkylation reaction. When this does occur, the alkyl group that is lost is usually a small group such as a methyl or ethyl group. Metabolic dealkylation is a reaction that is catalyzed by various members of the cytochrome P450 family of enzymes. In the most common cases of dealkylation of an ether, a phenol forms, which is then metabolized by the routes of metabolism open to phenol, namely the glucuronide or sulfate conjugation. The alkyl group is lost as an aldehyde, either formaldehyde (Fig. 8-4) or acetaldehyde if the alkyl radical is ethyl.

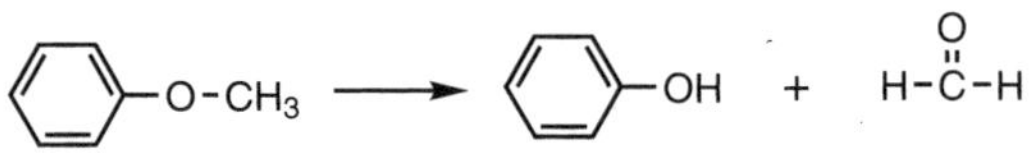

FIGURE 8-4. Metabolic dealkylation of anisole.

Aldehydes and Ketones

9

■ **NOMENCLATURE.** Two functional groups that, owing to their chemical and physical similarities, can be grouped together are the aldehydes and ketones. From the examples of common names shown in Figure 9-1, one can see that the structural identity of simple aldehydes and ketones is obvious since the term "aldehyde" or "ketone" appears in the nomenclature. The common nomenclature for aldehydes remains useful until one is unable to name the alkyl radical that contains the carbonyl, and then the formal IUPAC name is used. The longest continuous chain containing the aldehyde functional group is chosen as the base name and numbered such that the aldehyde constitutes the 1 position. To show the presence of an aldehyde in the molecule, the suffix "-al" replaces the "e" in the alkane base name. Hence, the more complex structure A shown in Figure 9-1 is named 3,3-dimethylbutanal.

With the common nomenclature of ketones, as indicated, the word "ketone" is used as part of the nomenclature. With ketones, the two radicals attached to the carbonyl are individually named until these radical names become unwieldy. The IUPAC rules for ketones require that one find the longest continuous carbon chain that contains the ketone and number so as to give the lowest number to the carbonyl group. If the ketone is at the same location from either end of the molecule, then the correct direction of numbering is the one that gives the lowest number to any remaining substituents. The designation used to show the presence of a ketone carbonyl is the suffix "-one" which, along with the ketone location, replaces the "e" in the alkane base name. The example given for structure B in Figure 9-1 becomes 2,5,7,7-tetramethyl-4-(the location of the carbonyl) octan (specifying an 8-carbon chain)-one (the abbreviation for a ketone).

■ **PHYSICAL-CHEMICAL PROPERTIES.** In considering the properties of aldehydes and ketones, it must be noted that the carbonyl group present in both molecules is polar, and hence the compounds are polar. Oxygen is more electronegative than carbon, and the cloud of electrons that makes up the carbon-oxygen double bond is therefore distorted toward the oxygen. In addition, ketones and to a lesser extent aldehydes may exist in equilibrium with the "enol" form (Fig. 9-2). This property and the polar nature of the carbonyl lead to higher boiling points for aldehydes and ketones compared with nonpolar compounds of comparable molecular weight. Because of the high electron density on the oxygen atom, aldehydes and ketones can hydrogen bond to water and will dissolve, to some extent, in water. The hydrogen bonding is similar to that suggested for ethers but stronger. Keep in mind that as the nonpolar hydrocarbon portion increases, the effect of the polar carbonyl

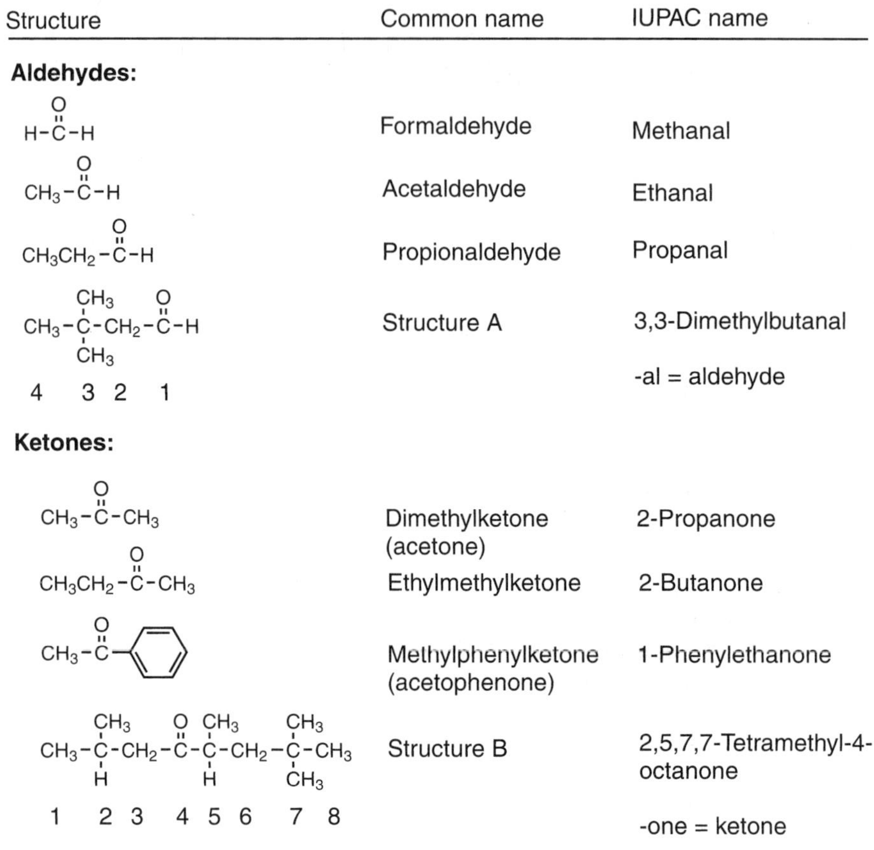

Structure	Common name	IUPAC name
Aldehydes:		
$\overset{\text{O}}{\overset{\|}{\text{H–C–H}}}$	Formaldehyde	Methanal
$\overset{\text{O}}{\overset{\|}{\text{CH}_3\text{–C–H}}}$	Acetaldehyde	Ethanal
$\overset{\text{O}}{\overset{\|}{\text{CH}_3\text{CH}_2\text{–C–H}}}$	Propionaldehyde	Propanal
$\text{CH}_3\text{–}\overset{\overset{\text{CH}_3}{\|}}{\underset{\underset{\text{CH}_3}{\|}}{\text{C}}}\text{–CH}_2\text{–}\overset{\text{O}}{\overset{\|}{\text{C}}}\text{–H}$ 4 3 2 1	Structure A	3,3-Dimethylbutanal
		-al = aldehyde
Ketones:		
$\overset{\text{O}}{\overset{\|}{\text{CH}_3\text{–C–CH}_3}}$	Dimethylketone (acetone)	2-Propanone
$\overset{\text{O}}{\overset{\|}{\text{CH}_3\text{CH}_2\text{–C–CH}_3}}$	Ethylmethylketone	2-Butanone
$\text{CH}_3\text{–}\overset{\text{O}}{\overset{\|}{\text{C}}}\text{–}\bigcirc$	Methylphenylketone (acetophenone)	1-Phenylethanone
$\text{CH}_3\text{–}\overset{\overset{\text{CH}_3}{\|}}{\underset{\underset{\text{H}}{\|}}{\text{C}}}\text{–CH}_2\text{–}\overset{\text{O}}{\overset{\|}{\text{C}}}\text{–}\overset{\overset{\text{CH}_3}{\|}}{\underset{\underset{\text{H}}{\|}}{\text{C}}}\text{–CH}_2\text{–}\overset{\overset{\text{CH}_3}{\|}}{\underset{\underset{\text{CH}_3}{\|}}{\text{C}}}\text{–CH}_3$ 1 2 3 4 5 6 7 8	Structure B	2,5,7,7-Tetramethyl-4-octanone
		-one = ketone

FIGURE 9-1. Aldehyde and ketone nomenclature.

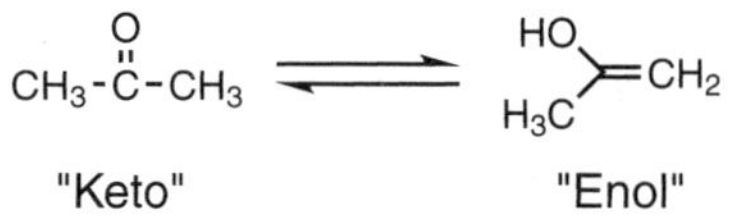

$$\overset{\text{O}}{\overset{\|}{\text{CH}_3\text{–C–CH}_3}} \rightleftharpoons \overset{\text{HO}}{\underset{\text{H}_3\text{C}}{>}}=\text{CH}_2$$

"Keto"   "Enol"

FIGURE 9-2. "Keto" - "enol" equilibrium of acetone.

group on overall solubility will decrease. This is illustrated in Table 9-1, where it is apparent that as the hydrocarbon portion increases beyond two or three carbons, the water solubility decreases rapidly in both aldehydes and ketones. Some water solubility is still possible, however, with a total carbon content of five or six carbons.

In considering the chemical reactivity from a pharmaceutical standpoint, the ketone functional group is relatively nonreactive. This is not true of the aldehyde functional group. Aldehydes are one oxidation state from the stable carboxylic acid

Table 9-1. BOILING POINTS AND WATER SOLUBILITY OF COMMON ALDEHYDES AND KETONES

	$\overset{\displaystyle O}{\overset{\|}{R-C-H}}$				$\overset{\displaystyle O}{\overset{\|}{R-C-R'}}$		
R	Boiling Point °C	Solubility (g/100g H$_2$O)	R	R'		Boiling Point °C	Solubility (g/100g H$_2$O)
H	-21	∞	CH$_3$	CH$_3$		56	∞
CH$_3$	20	∞	CH$_3$	C$_2$H$_5$		80	26.0
C$_2$H$_5$	49	16.0	CH$_3$	n-C$_3$H$_7$		102	6.3
n-C$_3$H$_7$	76	7.0	C$_2$H$_5$	C$_2$H$_5$		101	5.0
C$_6$H$_5$	178	0.3	C$_6$H$_5$	CH$_3$		202	<1.0

structure, and most are therefore rapidly oxidized. With many liquids, this means air oxidation, and compounds containing aldehydes therefore must be protected from atmospheric oxygen. The low-molecular-weight aldehydes can also undergo polymerization to cyclic trimers, a compound containing three aldehyde units, or straight-chain polymers (Fig. 9-3). The trimers are stable to oxygen but will allow regeneration of the aldehyde upon heating. In some cases, this reaction is used advantageously to protect the aldehyde.

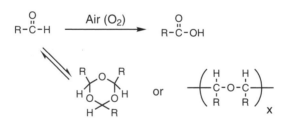

FIGURE 9-3. Oxidation and polymerization reactions of aldehydes.

A sequence of chemical reactions common to both aldehydes and ketones is the reaction that occurs between aldehydes or ketones and alcohols (Fig. 9-4). This reaction is catalyzed by acid. The reaction leading to hemiacetals or hemiketals and acetals or ketals is significant in that some drugs and many drug metabolites exist as one of these derivatives. The reaction of an aldehyde with an alcohol under acidic conditions gives a hemiacetal. "Hemi" refers to half, in this case half an acetal. The hemiacetal is unstable to aqueous conditions, irrespective of pH. Further addition of an alcohol to the hemiacetal can occur, leading to an acetal. Acetals are stable to

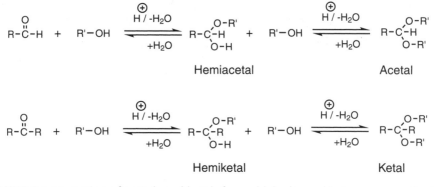

FIGURE 9-4. Formation of acetals and ketals from aldehydes and ketones, respectively.

aqueous conditions at neutral or basic pH but are unstable to aqueous acidic conditions, with conversion back to the aldehyde occurring. In a similar manner, a ketone may be converted to a hemiketal and further to a ketal by reaction with an alcohol under acidic conditions. The same stability properties exist for hemiketals and ketals as was mentioned for acetals. Probably the best examples of acetals are the glu-

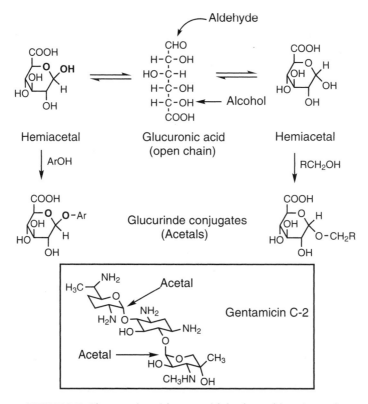

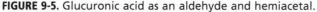

FIGURE 9-5. Glucuronic acid as an aldehyde and hemiacetal.

curonides formed between alcohols and phenols with glucuronic acid, while an example of an hemiacetal is the sugar glucuronic acid itself. In these cases the hemiacetal is an intramolecular hemiacetal (Fig. 9-5). The aminoglycoside antibiotics represent a drug class that possesses the acetal functional group, and the previously mentioned polymers of aldehydes are also examples of acetals.

■ **METABOLISM.** Several possible metabolic routes are found in vivo for aldehydes and ketones. Aldehydes in general are readily oxidized by xanthine oxidase, aldehyde oxidase, and NAD-specific aldehyde dehydrogenase, the resulting product being a carboxylic acid (Fig. 9-6). These oxidative enzymes are not cytochrome P450-associated enzymes.

A second metabolic reaction that may affect aldehydes and ketones is reduction. While reduction appears to be a minor metabolic reaction for aldehydes (Fig. 9-7), many ketones, especially α, β-unsaturated ketones, undergo reduction to a secondary alcohol. This reaction is often stereoselective, giving rise primarily to one isomer (Fig. 9-8).

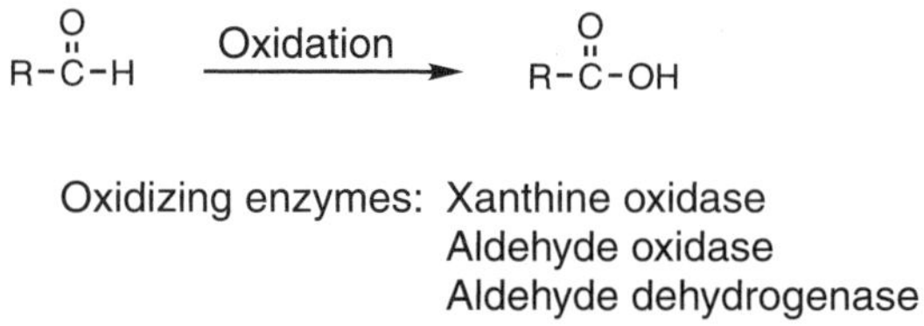

O
||
R–C–H   ⟶ Oxidation ⟶   R–C–OH
                              ||
                              O

Oxidizing enzymes: Xanthine oxidase
                    Aldehyde oxidase
                    Aldehyde dehydrogenase

FIGURE 9-6. Metabolic oxidation of aldehydes.

O
||
R–C–H   ⟶ Reduction ⟶   R–CH₂–OH

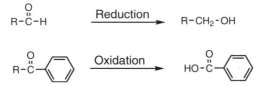

FIGURE 9-7. Minor metabolic reactions of aldehydes and ketones.

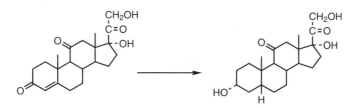

FIGURE 9-8. Metabolism of cortisone to tetrahydrocortisone.

Amines

10

AMINES—GENERAL

Two major functional groups still remain to be considered. These two groups, the carboxylic acids and the amines, are extremely important to medicinal chemistry and especially to the solubility nature of organic medicinals. In addition, the functional derivatives of these groups will be considered. In many instances the carboxylic acid or amine functional group is added to organic molecules with the specific purpose of promoting water solubility, since it is generally found that compounds showing little or no water solubility also are devoid of biologic activity.

■ **NOMENCLATURE.** The common nomenclature for amines is illustrated in Figure 10-1. Inspection of this nomenclature reveals that the common names consist of the name of the alkyl or aryl radical, followed by the word "amine." The examples given also show the different types of amines. The primary amine, isopropylamine, has a single substituent attached to the nitrogen; the secondary amine, ethylmethylamine, has two substituents attached to the nitrogen. The tertiary amine, t-butylethylmethylamine, has three groups attached directly to the nitrogen. As with all common nomenclatures, the system becomes nearly impossible to use as the branching of the alkyl groups increases, and the official nomen-

Structure	Common name (Alkylamine)	IUPAC name
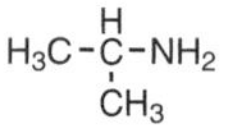 $H_3C-\overset{\overset{H}{\mid}}{\underset{\underset{CH_3}{\mid}}{C}}-NH_2$	Isopropylamine (Primary amine)	2-Aminopropane
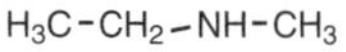 $H_3C-CH_2-NH-CH_3$	Ethylmethylamine (Secondary amine)	N-Methylaminoethane
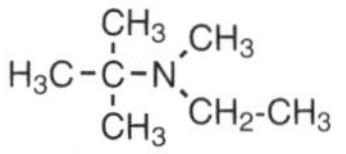 $H_3C-\overset{\overset{CH_3}{\mid}}{\underset{\underset{CH_3}{\mid}}{C}}-N\overset{CH_3}{\underset{CH_2-CH_3}{}}$	t-Butylethylmethylamine (Tertiary amine)	N-Ethyl-N-methyl-2-methyl-2-aminopropane
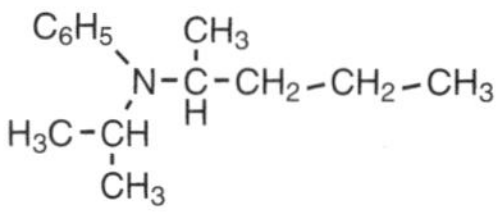 $\overset{C_6H_5}{\underset{H_3C-\underset{\mid}{CH}}{}}\overset{CH_3}{\underset{H}{N-\overset{\mid}{C}}}-CH_2-CH_2-CH_3$ $\underset{CH_3}{}$	N-Phenyl-N-(2-propyl)-2-aminopentane N = substituent on the Nitrogen	

FIGURE 10-1. Amine nomenclature.

clature becomes necessary. In the IUPAC system, the amines are considered substituted alkanes. The longest continuous alkyl chain containing the amine is identified and serves as the base name. The alkane chain is numbered in such a manner as to give the lowest possible number to the amine functional group, while the other substituents on the amine group are designated by use of a capital "N" before the name of the substituents. Examples are given in Figure 10-1.

■ **PHYSICAL-CHEMICAL PROPERTIES.** The amine functional group is probably one of the most common functional groups found in medicinal agents, and its value in the drug is twofold. One role is in solubilizing the drug either as the free base or as a water-soluble salt of the amine. The second role of the amine is to act as a binding site that holds the drug to a specific site in the body to produce the biologic activity. This latter role is beyond the scope of this book, but the former role contributes to an important physical property of the amine. First, let us pose a question: What influence will the amine functional group have on solubility properties? While amines are polar compounds, they may not show high boiling points or good water solubility. One reason for this is that in the tertiary amine, one does not find an electropositive group attached to the nitrogen. In the primary and secondary amines, one does have an electropositive hydrogen connected to the nitrogen, but the nitrogen is not as electronegative as oxygen, and the dipole is therefore weak. What all this means is that the amount of the intermolecular hydrogen bonding is minimal in primary and secondary amines and nonexistent in tertiary amines. This leads to relatively low-boiling liquids.

In considering water solubility, a different factor must be taken into account. The amine has an unshared pair of electrons, which leads to high electron density around the nitrogen. This high electron density promotes water solubility because hydrogen bonding between the hydrogen of water and the electron-dense nitrogen occurs. This is similar to the situation with low-molecular-weight ethers but occurs to a greater extent with basic amines. Both boiling points and the solubility effects are shown in Table 10-1. Also illustrated in Table 10-1 is the effect on solubility of increasing the hydrocarbon constituent. Primary amines tend to be more soluble than secondary amines, which are more soluble than tertiary amines. The amine can solubilize up to six or seven methylenes, which, from a solubility standpoint, makes the amines equivalent to an alcohol.

An extremely important property of the amines is their basicity and ability to form salts. The Brønsted definition of a base is the ability of a compound to accept a proton from an acid. Amines have an unshared pair of electrons, which is more or less available for sharing. The statement "more or less" has to do with the strength of a base, and this is considered in Figure 10-2. The strength of a base is defined by its relative ability to donate its unshared pair of electrons. The more readily the electrons are donated, the stronger the base. To define the strength of a base and to place this value on the same scale with acids, the measure of basicity of an amine is obtained by considering the acidity of the conjugate acid produced by protonating the amine. This protonation gives an ammonium ion and its dissociation constant is given as its pK_a. Therefore, a strong base is a substance that

Table 10-1. BOILING POINTS AND WATER SOLUBILITY OF COMMON AMINES

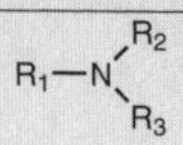

$$R_1-N\begin{smallmatrix}R_2\\\\R_3\end{smallmatrix}$$

R_1	R_2	R_3	Boiling Point °C	Solubility (g/100g H_2O)
CH_3	H	H	-7.5	very soluble
CH_3	CH_3	H	7.5	very soluble
CH_3	CH_3	CH_3	3.0	91
C_2H_5	H	H	17.0	miscible
C_2H_5	C_2H_5	H	55.0	very soluble
C_2H_5	C_2H_5	C_2H_5	89.0	14
C_6H_5	H	H	184	3.7
C_6H_5	CH_3	H	196	slightly soluble
C_6H_5	CH_3	CH_3	194	1.4

prefers to hold on to the proton, exist as the ammonium ion, and possess a small dissociation constant (K_a) and thus a large pK_a (Example 1). On the other hand, a weak base is a substance that does not readily donate its electrons and forms an unstable ammonium ion that dissociates readily with a large dissociation constant (K_a), and thus has a small pK_a (Example 2). Another way to view this relationship is that $pK_a = 14 - pK_b$. This may be of value since older references may define bases in terms of their K_b dissociation constant and the pK_b of a base.

Two factors influence basicity through the effects these factors have on the availability of the electrons. One of the factors is electronic, while the other is steric. To consider the former, if electron-donating groups are attached to the basic nitrogen, electrons are pushed into the nitrogen. Since a negative repels a negative, the elec-

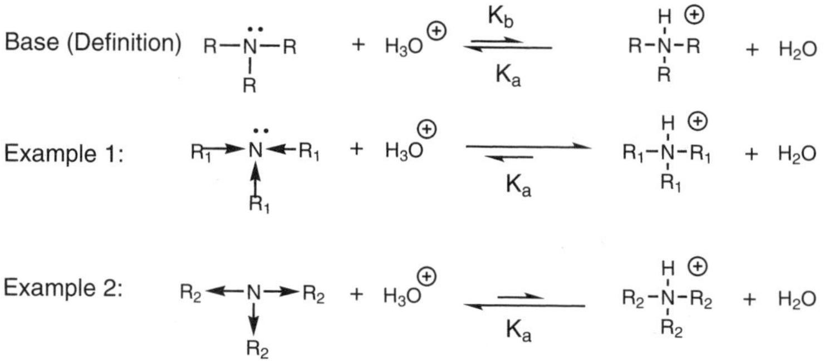

FIGURE 10-2. The influence of electron-releasing and electron-withdrawing groups on the basicity of amines.

tron pair on the nitrogen will be pushed out from the nitrogen, thus making the pair more readily available for donating.

If, on the other hand, electron-withdrawing or electron-attracting groups are attached to the nitrogen, the unshared pair of electrons will be pulled to the nitrogen atom and will be less readily available for donating, and therefore a weaker base results. An example of the electron donor is the alkyl, and an example of an electron-withdrawing group is the aryl or phenyl group. Based on this, one would predict that secondary alkyl amines with two electron-releasing groups attached to the nitrogen should be more basic than primary alkyl amines with a single alkyl group attached to the nitrogen. This is normally true. One would also predict that tertiary alkyl amines with three electron-releasing groups attached to the nitrogen should be more basic than secondary amines. This would be true if it were not for steric hindrance, the second factor that affects basicity. If large alkyl groups surround the unshared pair of electrons, then the approach of hydronium ions, a source of a proton, is hindered. The degree of this hindrance will affect the strength of basicity. The steric effect becomes important for tertiary amines but has little if any effect on primary and secondary amines. As shown in Figure 10-3, with amines, the large alkyl groups move back and forth, blocking the approach of water. Salt formation therefore does not occur as readily as it would in the absence of such hindrance. We commonly find that with alkyl amines, secondary amines are more basic than tertiary amines, and tertiary amines are more basic than primary amines.

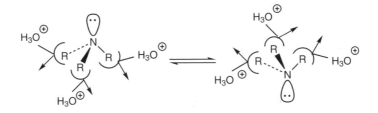

FIGURE 10-3. Diagrammatic representation of the influence of steric factors on the basicity of tertiary alkyl amines.

Aromatic amines differ significantly from alkyl amines in basicity. The aromatic ring, with its delocalized cloud of electrons, serves as an electron sink. The aromatic ring thus acts as an electron-withdrawing group, leading to a drop in basicity by six powers of ten. The unshared pair of electrons is said to be resonance stabilized, as shown in Figure 10-4. The spreading of the electron density over a greater area decreases the ability of the molecule to donate the electrons, and basicity is therefore reduced. Additional substitution on the nitrogen of aniline with an alkyl or a second aryl group changes the basicity in a predictable manner, with the alkyl group increasing basicity and an aryl reducing basicity to a nearly neutral compound (Table 10-2). Finally, substitution on the aromatic ring also affects basicity. Substitution meta or para to the amine has a predictable effect on

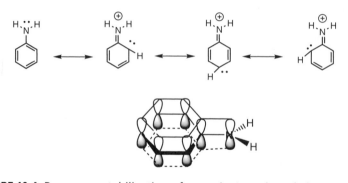

FIGURE 10-4. Resonance stabilization of an amine's unshared electron pair.

basicity, while ortho substitution affects basicity in an unpredictable manner (see Table 10-2). An electron-withdrawing group attached to the aromatic ring in the meta or para position decreases basicity. The decrease is significant if this group is para rather than meta. Electron-donating groups in the meta or para position usually increase basicity above that of aniline. The increase in basicity is most pronounced if the group is in the para position and not as pronounced if it is in the meta position. It will be noted that this is just the opposite of phenols. With ortho-substituted anilines, predictability fails because of intramolecular interactions.

Since amines are basic, one would expect that they react with acids to form salts. This is an important reaction, for if the salts that are formed dissociate in water, there is a strong likelihood that these salts will be water-soluble (Fig. 10-5). Such is the case with many organic drugs. If a basic amine is present in the drug, it can be converted into a salt, which in turn is used to prepare aqueous solutions of the drug. The most frequently used acids for preparing salts are hydrochloric, sulfuric, tartaric, succinic, citric, and maleic acids (Fig. 10-6). Hydrochloric acid is a monobasic acid; it has one proton and therefore reacts with one molecule of base. The others are dibasic acids (sulfuric, tartaric, succinic, and maleic) and tribasic acids (citric and phosphoric). The aqueous solution of the amine salt will have a characteristic pH that will vary depending on the acid used. The pH will be acidic when a strong mineral acid is used to prepare the salt or weakly acidic or neutral if a weak organic acid is used. Since the amine is converted to a water-soluble salt by the action of the acid, it is reasonable to assume that the addition of a base to the

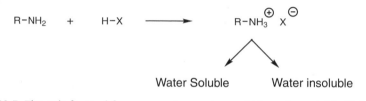

FIGURE 10-5. The salt formed from an amine and an acid is water soluble if the salt is able to dissociate and is water insoluble if the salt is unable to dissociate.

Table 10-2. PKA VALUES IN WATER OF COMMON PROTONATED AMINES

$$R_1\!-\!\overset{R_2}{\underset{R_3}{N}}\!-\!H \oplus + H_2O \overset{k_a}{\rightleftharpoons} R_1\!-\!N\overset{R_2}{\underset{R_3}{\diagdown}} + H_3O \oplus$$

R_1	R_2	R_3	pka
CH_3	H	H	10.62
CH_3CH_2	H	H	10.64
$(CH_3)_3C$	H	H	10.68
$CH_3(CH_2)_2$	H	H	10.58
CH_3	CH_3	H	10.71
CH_3CH_2	CH_3CH_2	H	10.92
$CH_3(CH_2)_2$	$CH_3(CH_2)_2$	H	10.91
CH_3	CH_3	CH_3	9.78
CH_3CH_2	CH_3CH_2	CH_3CH_2	10.75
C_6H_5	H	H	4.62
C_6H_5	CH_3	H	4.85
$p\text{-}O_2N\text{-}C_6H_4$	H	H	1.00
$m\text{-}O_2N\text{-}C_6H_4$	H	H	2.51
$p\text{-}Cl\text{-}C_6H_4$	H	H	3.98
$m\text{-}Cl\text{-}C_6H_4$	H	H	3.52
$p\text{-}CH_3\text{-}C_6H_4$	H	H	5.08
$m\text{-}CH_3\text{-}C_6H_4$	H	H	4.69
$p\text{-}CH_3O\text{-}C_6H_4$	H	H	5.34
$m\text{-}CH_3O\text{-}C_6H_4$	H	H	4.23
C_6H_5	C_6H_5	H	0.85

salt would result in liberation of the free amine, which in turn may precipitate. This is a chemical incompatibility that could be quite important when drugs are mixed. Included in Figure 10-6 are two additional commonly used acids, pamoic and hydroxynaphthoic acid. These acids are commonly used in medicinal chemistry to form amine salts that are water-insoluble (in other words, salts that will not disso-

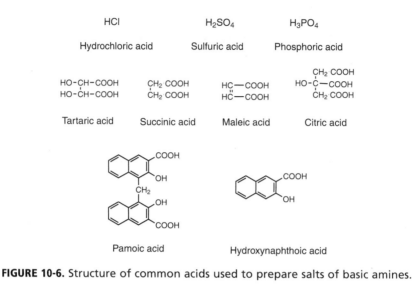

FIGURE 10-6. Structure of common acids used to prepare salts of basic amines.

ciate). This property is used to good advantage in that it prevents a drug from being absorbed and thus keeps the drug in the intestinal tract.

■ **METABOLISM.** Many metabolic routes are available for handling amines in the body, some of which are illustrated in Figure 10-7. A common reaction that secondary and tertiary amines undergo is dealkylation. In the dealkylation reaction, the alkyl group is lost as an aldehyde or ketone and the amine is converted from a tertiary amine to a secondary amine and finally to a primary amine. This reaction usually occurs when the amine is substituted with small alkyl groups such as a methyl, ethyl, or propyl group. An example of a drug metabolized by a dealkylation reaction is imipramine, which is metabolized to desimipramine. These dealkylation reactions are commonly catalyzed by members of the cytochrome P450 family of enzymes.

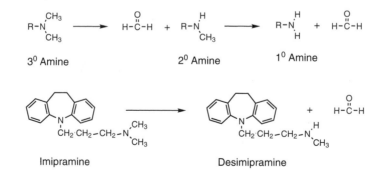

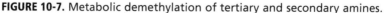

FIGURE 10-7. Metabolic demethylation of tertiary and secondary amines.

Primary alkyl amines can also undergo a dealkylation reaction of sorts known as deamination. Here again, an aldehyde or ketone is formed along with an amine. Pyridoxal 5-phosphate may catalyze this reaction, resulting in the formation of pyridoxamine. For this reaction to occur, a carbon bonded to the nitrogen must be substituted with at least one hydrogen. The enzymes most commonly found that catalyze deamination reactions are monoamine oxidase (MAO) and diamine oxidase (DAO). An example of an MAO-catalyzed reaction is the deamination of norepinephrine, as shown in Figure 10-8. MAO is not a cytochrome P450 enzyme, although under some circumstances primary amines may undergo a CYP450-catalyzed dealkylation.

A minor metabolic route open to amines is the methylation reaction. An important example of the methylation reaction is the biosynthesis of epinephrine from norepinephrine by the enzyme phenylethanolamine-N-methyltransferase (Fig. 10-9).

Far more important to the metabolism of primary and secondary, but not tertiary, amines are the conjugation reactions. Amines can be conjugated with glucuronic acid and sulfuric acid to give the glucuronides and sulfates, both of which

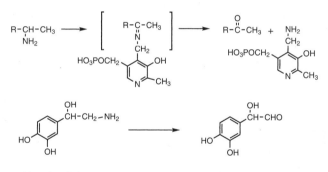

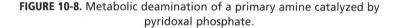

Norepinephrine

FIGURE 10-8. Metabolic deamination of a primary amine catalyzed by pyridoxal phosphate.

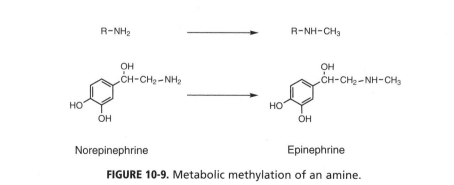

R–NH₂ is shown as $R-NH_2$ transforming to $R-NH-CH_3$.

Norepinephrine   Epinephrine

FIGURE 10-9. Metabolic methylation of an amine.

exhibit a significant increase in water solubility. Amines, especially primary aryl amines, may also be acetylated by acetyl CoA to give a compound that usually shows a decrease in water solubility (Fig. 10-10). Conjugation reactions are considered phase 2 metabolic reactions (see Appendix C).

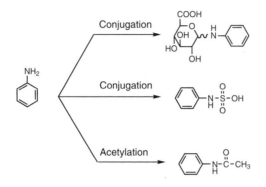

FIGURE 10-10. Metabolic conjugation of a primary amine with glucuronic acid, sulfuric acid, and acetyl coenzyme A (Phase 2 conjugations).

QUATERNARY AMMONIUM SALTS

Special amine derivatives with unique properties are the quaternary ammonium salts.

■ **NOMENCLATURE.** While the reaction of primary, secondary, or tertiary amines with acid leads to the formation of the respective ammonium salts, these reactions can be reversed by treatment with base, regenerating the initial amines (Fig. 10-11). The quaternary ammonium salts we wish to consider here are those compounds in which the nitrogen is bound to four carbon atoms through covalent bonds.

The quaternary ammonium salts are stable compounds that are not converted to amines by treatment with base. The nitrogen-carbon bonds may be alkyl bonds, aryl bonds, or a mixture of alkyl-aryl bonds. The nomenclature is derived by naming the organic substituents, followed by the word "ammonium" and then the particular salt that is present. An example is the compound tetraethyl ammonium (TEA) sulfate:

$$\left(C_2H_5 - \overset{\overset{\displaystyle C_2H_5}{|}}{\underset{\underset{\displaystyle C_2H_5}{|}}{N}} \!\!-\! C_2H_5 \right)_2^{\oplus} SO_4^{2-}$$

TEA Sulfate

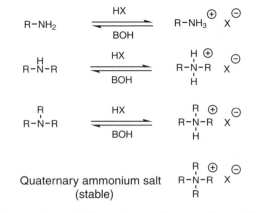

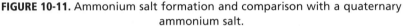

FIGURE 10-11. Ammonium salt formation and comparison with a quaternary ammonium salt.

■ **PHYSICAL-CHEMICAL PROPERTIES.** Although the ammonium salts formed from primary, secondary, and tertiary amines are reversible, as shown in Figure 10-11, this is not true of quaternary ammonium salts. These salts are relatively stable and require considerable energy to break the carbon-nitrogen bond. The quaternary ammonium salts are ionic compounds that, if capable of dissociation in water, exhibit significant water solubility. Ion-dipole bonding to water of the quaternary ammonium has the potential of dissolving 20 to 30 carbon atoms. Most of the quaternary ammonium salts commonly seen in pharmacy are water-soluble.

■ **METABOLISM.** There is no special metabolism of quaternary ammonium salts that the student need be familiar with.

Carboxylic Acids

11

■ **NOMENCLATURE—COMMON AND IUPAC NOMENCLATURE.** A carboxylic acid is a molecule that contains a characteristic carboxyl group to which is attached a hydrogen, alkyl, aryl, or heterocyclic substituent. The common nomenclature of the carboxylic acids is used more often than with most other functional groups, probably because of the wide variety of carboxylic acids found in nature and the fact that they were named before the chemistry of the molecules was understood. Even without branching of the alkyl chains, this nomenclature becomes difficult to remember, with such uncommon names as caproic (C_6), caprylic (C_8), capric (C_{10}), and lauric (C_{12}) acids. The official nomenclature returns to the use of the hydrocarbon names such as methane, ethane, propane, butane, and pentane. As with all IUPAC nomenclature, the longest continuous chain containing the functional group, in this case the carboxyl group, is chosen as the base unit. The hydrocarbon name is used, the "e" is dropped and replaced with "oic," which signifies a carboxyl group, and this is followed by the word "acid." This is illustrated in Figure 11-1.

Structure	Common name	IUPAC name
O‖ H–C–OH	Formic acid	Methan<u>oic</u> acid
O‖ CH$_3$–C–OH	Acetic acid (vinegar)	Ethan<u>oic</u> acid
O‖ CH$_3$–CH$_2$–C–OH	Propionic acid	Propan<u>oic</u> acid
O‖ CH$_3$–CH$_2$–CH$_2$–CH$_2$–CH$_2$–C–OH	Caproic acid	Hexan<u>oic</u> acid
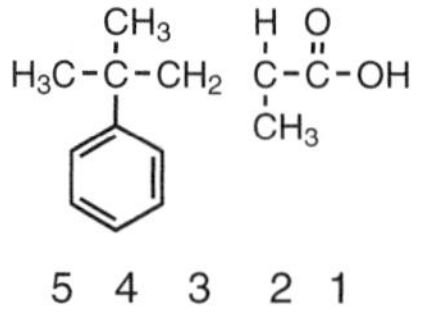 CH$_3$ H O‖ H$_3$C–C–CH$_2$ C–C–OH (phenyl) CH$_3$ 5 4 3 2 1	2,4-Dimethyl-4-phenylpentan<u>oic</u> acid	

FIGURE 11-1. Examples of Common and Official (IUPAC) nomenclature for carboxylic acids.

■ **NOMENCLATURE—BIOLOGICALLY IMPORTANT CARBOXYLIC ACIDS.** The student should be familiar with a number of biologically significant carboxylic acids related to drug actions and nutrition. Mevalonic acid, one such compound, is a key intermediate in the biosynthesis of cholesterol, which itself serves as the precursor to most of the steroid hormones in the human body.

Mevalonic acid
(3,5-Dihydroxy-3-
methylpentanoic acid)   - - - - - ▶ Squalene - - - - - ▶ Steroids
                                                          (Cholesterol)

Important in human nutrition are the naturally occurring carboxylic acids known as the fatty acids. These compounds derive their name from the physico-chemical property of being quite fat-soluble, thus the terminology of fatty acids. Included within this group are the acids lauric, myristic, palmitic, and stearic acid (Table 11-1). These acids all have an even number of carbons, which relates to their common biosynthetic pathway in which two carbon acetate units are linked to form the naturally occurring fatty acids. In addition, these acids are all saturated fatty acids, a form of nomenclature used in identifying fat content on food labels. The

Table 11-1. BOILING POINTS (BP)/MELTING POINTS (MP) AND WATER SOLUBILITY OF COMMON ORGANIC ACIDS

Carboxylic acid	$R\text{-}\overset{O}{\overset{\|}{C}}\text{-}OH$	bp/mp ^0C	Solubility (g/100g H_2O)	(g/100g EtOH)
Formic	H	100.5	∞	∞
Acetic	CH_3	118.0	∞	∞
Propionic	CH_3CH_2	141.0	∞	∞
Butyric	$CH_3(CH_2)_2$	164.0	∞	∞
Pentanoic	$CH_3(CH_2)_3$	187.0	3.7	Soluble
Hexanoic	$CH_3(CH_2)_4$	205.0	1.0	Soluble
Benzoic	C_6H_5	250.0	0.34	Soluble
Decanoic	$CH_3(CH_2)_8$	31.4	0.015	Soluble
Lauric	$CH_3(CH_2)_{10}$	44	Insoluble	100
Myristic	$CH_3(CH_2)_{12}$	58.5	Insoluble	Soluble
Palmitic	$CH_3(CH_2)_{14}$	63-64	Insoluble	Sparingly
Stearic	$CH_3(CH_2)_{16}$	69-70	Insoluble	5.0

term "saturated" refers to the fact that all the carbons, with the exception of the carboxylic acid group, are fully saturated with hydrogen. Palmitic and stearic acids are the most abundant of the saturated fatty acids.

A second group of fatty acids are the monounsaturated fatty acids. The most common members of this class of agents are palmitoleic acid and oleic acid. A common feature of the monounsaturated fatty acids is that the double bond is usually found at the nine position (Δ^9) and is "cis" in stereochemistry.

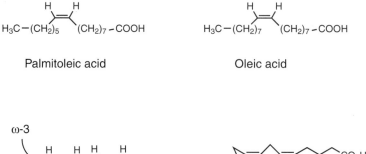

Palmitoleic acid   Oleic acid

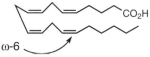

Linoleic acid   Arachidonic acid

A third group of fatty acids are the polyunsaturated fatty acids. By definition, polyunsaturated suggests two or more double bonds. The most common polyunsaturated fatty acids are linolenic, linoleic, and arachidonic acid which are also known as the omega fatty acids (the first is ω-3 and the latter two are ω-6). The omega nomenclature indicates that a double bond is found either three carbons from the terminal methyl group or six carbons from the terminal methyl group, respectively. Linoleic and linolenic acid are commonly referred to as the "essential

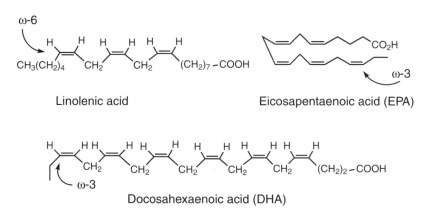

Linolenic acid   Eicosapentaenoic acid (EPA)

Docosahexaenoic acid (DHA)

fatty acids" in that they are essential for the synthesis of cell membranes as well as other functions in the body. Arachidonic acid is a key intermediate in the biosynthesis of the prostaglandin, prostacyclin, and thromboxane hormones (Fig. 11-2).

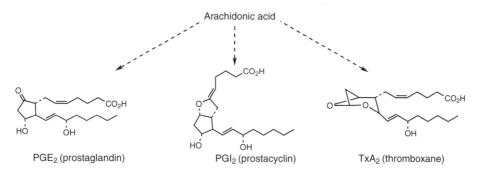

FIGURE 11-2. Biosynthesis of prostaglandins, postacyclins, and thromboxanes from acachidonic acid.

Most recently, several dietary fish oils have been identified as having significant effects in reducing coronary artery disease. Examples of important fish oils are EPA (a precursor to prostaglandin-3) and DHA.

■ **PHYSICAL-CHEMICAL PROPERTIES.** The carboxylic acid functional group consists of a carbonyl and a hydroxyl group; both, when taken individually, are polar groups that can hydrogen bond. The hydrogen of the -OH can hydrogen bond to either of the oxygen groups in another carboxyl function (Fig. 11-3). The amount and strength of hydrogen bonding in the case of a carboxylic acid are greater than in the case of alcohols or phenols because of the greater acidity of the carboxylic acid and because of the additional sites of bonding. From this discussion, one could predict that carboxylic acids are high-boiling liquids and solids. If the carboxyl can strongly hydrogen bond to itself, then it is reasonable to predict that the carboxyl group can hydrogen bond to water, resulting in water solubility. In Table 11-1, the effect of the strong intermolecular hydrogen bonding can be seen by examining the boiling points of several of the carboxylic acids, while the strong hydrogen bonding to water is demonstrated by the solubility of the carboxylic acids in water. Once again, as the lipophilic hydrocarbon chain length increases, the water solubility decreases

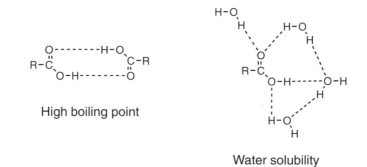

FIGURE 11-3. Intermolecular bonding of carboxylic acids to themselves and to water.

drastically. A carboxyl group will solubilize (1% or greater concentration) approximately five carbon atoms.

Another solvent important in pharmacy is ethanol. Ethanol has both a hydrophilic and lipophilic portion, and bonding between an organic molecule and ethanol therefore may involve both dipole-dipole bonding and van der Waals bonding. It is not surprising, then, that the solubility of the carboxylic acids is much greater in ethanol than it is in water. Although pure ethanol cannot be used internally, ethanol-water combinations can, and they greatly increase the solution potential of many drugs.

Turning now to an extremely important property of the carboxylic acids, their acidic property, one sees the familiar dissociation of a carboxylic acid (giving up a proton) shown in Table 11-2. This dissociation, by definition, makes the group an acid.

From general chemistry it will be recalled that the strength of an acid depends on the concentration of protons in solution, which depends on dissociation. The

Table 11-2. DISSOCIATION CONSTANTS AND pK$_a$ VALUES IN WATER OF COMMON CARBOXYLIC ACIDS

$R-C-OH$	K_a (in water)	pK_a
H	17.7×10^{-5}	3.75
CH_3	1.75×10^{-5}	4.76
$Cl-CH_2$	1.36×10^{-3}	2.87
Cl_2CH	5.53×10^{-2}	1.26
Cl_3C	2.32×10^{-1}	0.64
C_6H_5	6.30×10^{-5}	4.21
p -CH_3-C_6H_4	4.20×10^{-5}	4.38
m - CH_3-C_6H_4	5.40×10^{-5}	4.27
P - NO_2-C_6H_4	3.60×10^{-4}	3.44
m - NO_2-C_6H_4	3.20×10^{-4}	3.50

value of K_1 and K_{-1} in turn depends on the stability of the carboxylate anion in relation to the undissociated carboxylic acid. In other words, if we are considering two acids, acid 1 (in which the carboxylate anion is unstable) and acid 2 (in which the carboxylate anion is stable), acid 2, with the more stable carboxylate, will dissociate to a greater extent, giving up a higher concentration of protons, and therefore is a stronger acid. It has been found that the nature of the R-group *does* influence the stability of the carboxylate anion, and it does so in the following manner: if R is an electron donor group, as shown in Table 11-2, it will destabilize the carboxylate anion and thus decrease the acidity (this is represented by the dissociation arrows). To understand how this comes about, one must look at the carboxylate anion. This anion is stabilized by resonance, with the negative charge not remaining fixed on the oxygen but instead being spread across the oxygen-carbon-oxygen. Now, if electrons are pushed toward a region already high in electron density, repulsion occurs. This is an unfavorable situation. In the nonionic carboxylic acid form, resonance stabilization is not occurring to the same extent and the problem is reduced. Therefore, in Example 1, the nonionic form is more stable than the ionic form. In Example 2, the opposite effect is considered: electron withdrawal by the R-group. Reducing electron density around the carbonyl carbon should increase the ease of resonance stabilization, in turn increasing the stability of the carboxylate anion. Considering Example 2 in relationship to Example 1, one would predict that acid 2 would be more acidic than acid 1. Table 11-2 has examples of compounds that fit this description. The methyl group is an electron donor that reduces the acidity with respect to that of formic acid, while the phenyl can be considered an electron sink or, with respect to alkyl acids, an electron-withdrawing group; therefore, benzoic acid is a stronger acid than acetic acid. The addition of halogens to an alkyl changes the nature of the alkyl. In chloroacetic acid, the chloride, being electronegative, pulls electrons away from the carbon, which in turn pulls electrons away from the carbonyl. This effect is quite strong, as is seen in the K_a. This electron-withdrawing effect continues to increase as the number of halogens increases to give a strong carboxylic acid, trichloroacetic acid.

As discussed earlier for phenols and aromatic amines, substitution on the aromatic ring of benzoic acid will influence acidity. Ortho substitution is not always predictable, but in most cases the acidity of the acid is increased by ortho substitution. Meta and para substitutions are predictable. Substitution on the benzene ring with an electron-releasing group decreases acidity. If this substituent is para, the decrease in acidity with respect to benzoic acid will be greater than if the substituent is meta. If the substituent is an electron-withdrawing group, the acidity of the acid will increase. The greatest increase is observed when the substituent is para. One should recall that this is the same trend seen for substituted phenols.

Another property of carboxylic acids is their reactivity toward base. Carboxylic acids will react with a base to give a salt, as shown in Table 11-3. If one is considering water solubility, the interaction of a salt with water through dipole-ion bonding is much stronger than dipole-dipole interaction of the acid. Therefore, a considerable increase in water solubility should and does occur. The same point must be made here as was made with phenol and amine salts: the salt must be able to

Table 11-3. SOLUBILITY PROPERTIES OF SODIUM SALTS OF COMMON ORGANIC ACIDS

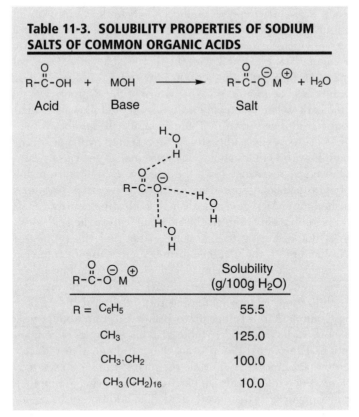

$R-\overset{O}{\underset{}{C}}-O^{\ominus} M^{\oplus}$	Solubility (g/100g H_2O)
R = C_6H_5	55.5
CH_3	125.0
$CH_3 \cdot CH_2$	100.0
$CH_3 (CH_2)_{16}$	10.0

dissociate in order to dissolve in water. Salts formed from carboxylic acids and sodium, potassium, or ammonium hydroxide show a great increase in water solubility. Salts formed with heavy metals tend to be relatively insoluble. Examples of such insoluble salts are the heavy metal salts (e.g., calcium, magnesium, zinc, aluminium) of carboxylic acids. When salts of carboxylic acids dissolve in water, a characteristic alkaline pH is common. With sodium and potassium salts, the pH is generally quite high. As with other salts, if acid is now added to this solution, one can reverse the carboxylic acid-base reaction and regenerate the carboxylic acid. The free acid is less soluble than was the salt, and precipitation may result. This is an important chemical incompatibility that one should keep in mind when dealing with water-soluble carboxylate salts. In summary, amines and carboxylic acids are common functional groups found in drugs. These groups have a potentiating effect on solubility, and both groups can form salts that, if capable of dissociation, will greatly increase water solubility.

■ **METABOLISM.** The metabolism of the carboxylic acids is relatively simple. Carboxylic acids can undergo a variety of conjugation reactions (phase 2 metabolism; see Appendix C). They can conjugate with glucuronic acid to form glu-

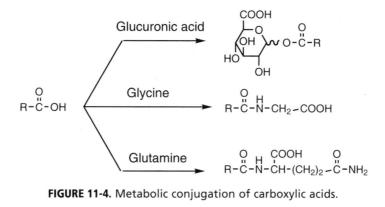

FIGURE 11-4. Metabolic conjugation of carboxylic acids.

curonides and also with amino acids (Fig. 11-4). Glycine and glutamine are two common amino acids that form conjugates with acids.

Another common type of metabolism of alkyl carboxylic acids is oxidation beta to the carboxyl group. This is a common reaction in the metabolism of fatty acids. The reaction proceeds through a sequence in which the carboxyl group is bound to coenzyme A (CoA). The bound acid is oxidized to enoyl CoA, hydrated to β-hydroxyacetyl CoA, oxidized to β-ketoacyl CoA, and finally cleaved to the shortened carboxylic acid plus acetic acid, as shown in Figure 11-5.

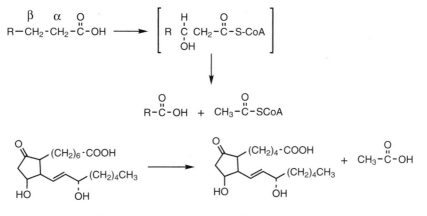

FIGURE 11-5. Beta oxidation of alkyl carboxylic acids.

Functional Derivatives of Carboxylic Acids

12

In presenting the carboxylic acids, it is important to also consider several derivatives of carboxylic acids. The first to be discussed will be the esters.

ESTERS

■ **NOMENCLATURE.** The nomenclature consists of combining the alcohol and carboxylic acid nomenclature as either common nomenclature or as IUPAC nomenclature, but not mixed. The name of the alcohol radical comes first, followed by a space, and then the name of the acid. To show that it is a functional derivative of an acid, the "ic" ending of the acid is dropped and replaced by "ate." Examples are shown in Figure 12-1. If you do not remember alcohol and acid nomenclature, you should return to the appropriate sections and review this material.

A unique type of ester results from the intramolecular cyclization of an alcohol and a carboxylic acid. The resulting ester is known as a lactone (Fig. 12-2). Lactones are quite common in drug molecules and may exist with a five- (spironolactone) or six- (testolactone) membered ring up to and exceeding 14-unit rings (macrolide antibiotics such as erythromycin). The physical-chemical and metabolic properties of a lactone are the same as those of an ester.

■ **PHYSICAL-CHEMICAL PROPERTIES.** The physical properties of the esters are rather interesting and show a similarity to the ethers. In the formation of esters, a polar alcohol is combined with a polar acid to give a much less polar, low-boiling liquid. In the case of ethers, two alcohols are joined with the same decrease in polarity and boiling points. As with ethers, in the ester, the two hydroxyl groups

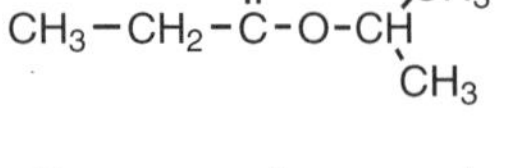

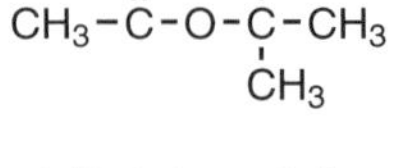

$$CH_3-CH_2-\overset{\overset{\displaystyle O}{\|}}{C}-O-CH\overset{\displaystyle CH_3}{\underset{\displaystyle CH_3}{}}$$

$$CH_3-\overset{\overset{\displaystyle O}{\|}}{C}-O-\overset{\overset{\displaystyle CH_3}{|}}{\underset{\displaystyle CH_3}{C}}-CH_3$$

Common: Isopropyl propion<u>ate</u>   t-Butyl acet<u>ate</u>

IUPAC   : 2-Propyl propano<u>ate</u>   2-Methyl-2-propyl ethano<u>ate</u>

FIGURE 12-1. Examples of Common and Official (IUPAC) nomenclature of esters.

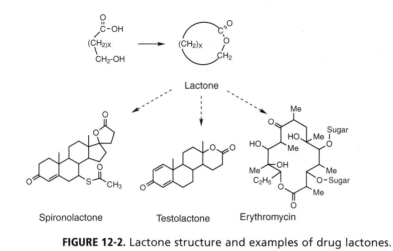

FIGURE 12-2. Lactone structure and examples of drug lactones.

necessary for intermolecular hydrogen bonding are destroyed, and along with this goes the loss of the intermolecular hydrogen bonding and a decrease in water solubility. Proof of this effect can be seen in Table 12-1. The boiling point of acetic acid is 118°, which itself is above that of many of the esters. The water solubility of esters is due to hydrogen bonding between the hydrogen of water and the electron-dense oxygen of the ester carbonyl. While esters are not highly water-soluble, they are quite soluble in alcohol.

Table 12-1. BOILING POINTS AND WATER SOLUBILITY OF COMMON ESTERS

$$R-\overset{\overset{\displaystyle O}{\|}}{C}-O-R'$$

R	R'	Boiling Point °C	Solubility (g/100g H$_2$O)
CH$_3$	CH$_3$	57.5	∞
CH$_3$	CH$_3$CH$_2$	77.0	10.0
CH$_3$CH$_2$	CH$_3$	79.7	6.25
CH$_3$	CH$_3$CH$_2$CH$_2$	102.0	1.60
CH$_3$	CH$_3$CH$_2$CH$_2$CH$_2$	126.0	0.83
CH$_3$(CH$_2$)$_2$	CH$_3$	102.0	1.67
C$_6$H$_5$	CH$_3$	198.0	Insoluble

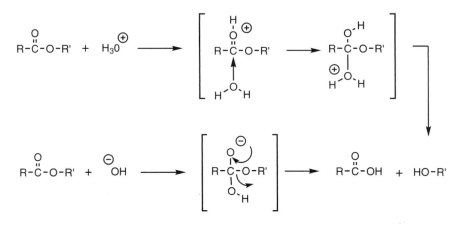

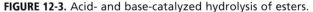

FIGURE 12-3. Acid- and base-catalyzed hydrolysis of esters.

An important chemical property that most esters display is the ease of hydrolysis back to the alcohol and the carboxylic acid. Esters are especially prone to base-catalyzed hydrolysis but also hydrolyze in the presence of acid and water (Fig. 12-3). What this means to medicinal chemistry is that esters are unstable in the presence of basic media in vitro and must therefore be protected from strongly alkaline conditions.

■ **METABOLISM.** Hydrolyzing enzymes in the body carry out hydrolysis through a base-catalyzed mechanism. It is therefore not unexpected that esters are unstable in the body and are converted to the free acid and the alcohol (Fig. 12-4). In many cases, carboxylic acids are synthetically prepared and administered as esters, even though the active drug is the acid. It is known that the acid will be regenerated metabolically.

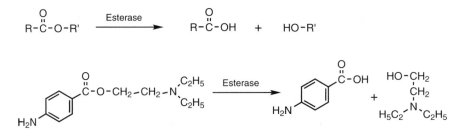

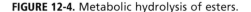

FIGURE 12-4. Metabolic hydrolysis of esters.

AMIDES

◼ **NOMENCLATURE.** The second important functional derivative of the carboxylic acid is the amide. An example of the common and official nomenclature is shown in Figure 12-5. In the case of the common nomenclature, the common name of the amine followed by the common name of the acid is used. The ending "ic" of the acid is then dropped and replaced by "amide." The same approach is used for official nomenclature except that the official name of the amine and the official name of the acid are used. The "oic" ending is dropped and replaced by "amide."

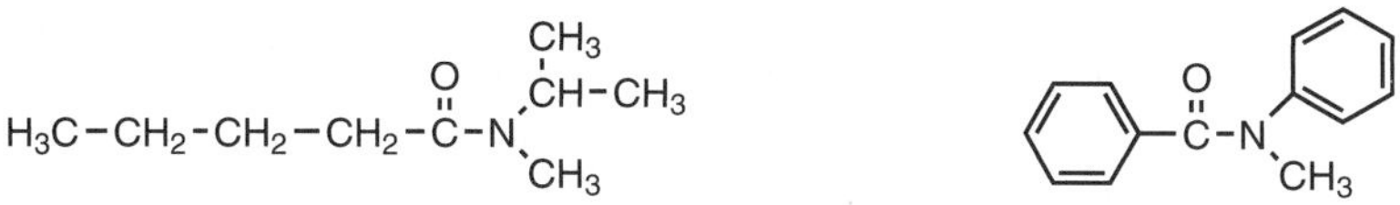

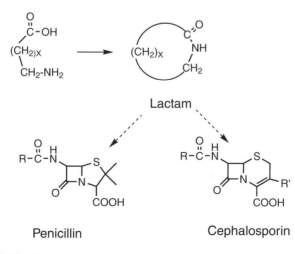

Common: N-Methyl-N-isopropyl valer<u>amide</u>   N-Methyl-N-phenyl benz<u>amide</u>

IUPAC   : N-Methyl-N-2-propyl pentan<u>amide</u>   N-Methyl-N-phenylbenz<u>amide</u>

FIGURE 12-5. Examples of Common and Official (IUPAC) nomenclature of amides.

A unique type of amide results from the intramolecular cyclization of an amine and a carboxylic acid. The resulting amide is known as a lactam (Fig. 12-6). As with the lactones, lactams make up the nucleus of several classes of important drugs. Probably the best-known lactam drugs are the β-lactams, which are found in the penicillins and cephalosporin antibiotics. The lactams possess physical-chemical

FIGURE 12-6. Lactam structure and examples of drug lactams.

and metabolic characteristics similar to those of the open chain amides, although with small ring compounds, such as the β-lactams, a high order of reactivity is seen.

■ **PHYSICAL-CHEMICAL PROPERTIES AND METABOLISM.** The physical properties of the amides are much different than might have been predicted after the earlier discussions of esters. Like the esters, the amides have a polar carboxylic acid combined with the weakly polar primary or secondary amine or ammonia to give the monosubstituted, disubstituted, or unsubstituted amides, respectively. The resulting amides still possess considerable polarity, as indicated by the high boiling points and water solubility (Table 12-2). These properties are quite different from those of esters. It is interesting to note that, with any series, as the substitution on the nitrogen increases, the boiling point decreases. As an example, look at formamide, N-methyl formamide, and N,N-dimethylformamide. This may be explained in part by a consideration of the resonance forms of amides, as shown in Figure 12-7. The unshared pair of electrons of the nitrogen no longer remain on the nitrogen but are spread across the nitrogen, carbon, and oxygen. This has a significant effect on the polarity of the amide. Since boiling points depend on the amount and strength of intermolecular bonding, the unsubstituted and monosubstituted amide would be expected to show strong intermolecular bonding owing to the high electron density on oxygen bonding to the hydrogens or hydrogen on the nitrogen. In the case of the disubstituted amides, both hydrogens have been replaced on the nitrogen, and intermolecular hydrogen bonding is not possible. Disubstituted amides are still

Table 12-2. BOILING POINTS AND WATER SOLUBILITY OF COMMON AMIDES

$$R_1-\overset{\overset{\displaystyle O}{\|}}{C}-N\overset{\displaystyle R_2}{\underset{\displaystyle R_3}{}}$$

R_1	R_2	R_3	Boiling Point ^{0}C	Solubility (g/100g H_2O)
H	H	H	210	Soluble
H	CH_3	H	180	Soluble
H	CH_3	CH_3	153	Soluble
CH_3	H	H	222	200
CH_3	CH_3	H	210	Soluble
CH_3	CH_3	CH_3	163	Soluble
C_6H_5	H	H	288	1.35
H	C_6H_5	H	271	2.86
CH_3	C_6H_5	H	304	0.53

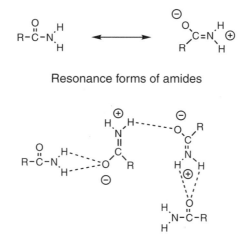

Resonance forms of amides

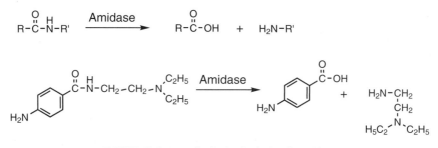

FIGURE 12-7. The effect of resonance structures of amides on intermolecular hydrogen bonding.

capable of dipole-dipole bonding, but not through hydrogen bonding. Thus, the boiling point drops. Water solubility requires only a polar material, since the hydrogen can be supplied by the water. Both substituted and unsubstituted amides can hydrogen bond to water through the hydrogen of water and show good water solubility. As the hydrocarbon portion of the amide increases, so the lipophilic nature increases and water solubility decreases.

A chemical property that differentiates amides from esters is the greater stability of the amide. Amides are relatively stable to the acid, base, and enzymatic conditions encountered in pharmacy. The reason for this stability again can be related to the resonance forms of the amide with its overlapping clouds of electrons. The importance of the increase in stability of the amide over the ester has been used to advantage in preparing drugs with prolonged activity. Although amides are relatively stable to acid, base, and enzymes, metabolic hydrolysis can occur, catalyzed by the amidase enzymes. An example is illustrated in Figure 12-8. The important point to remember is that amides are more stable in vivo than are esters.

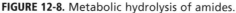

FIGURE 12-8. Metabolic hydrolysis of amides.

Although basic amines were used to prepare the amides, amides are nearly neutral functional groups, and therefore acid salts cannot be formed. Returning to the definition of a base, an unshared pair of electrons is essential for basicity. The unshared pair of electrons must be available for donation, a situation that does not exist in amides. In the amide, the pair of electrons no longer remain on the nitrogen but are spread over the nitrogen, carbon, and the oxygen. This resonance of the electrons reduces their availability and thus the amide's basicity.

CARBONATES, CARBAMATES, AND UREAS

The next functional derivatives of the carboxylic acids will be grouped together because of their similarity to the previously discussed esters and amides. The carbonates, carbamates, and ureas, functional derivatives of carbonic acid, are shown below.

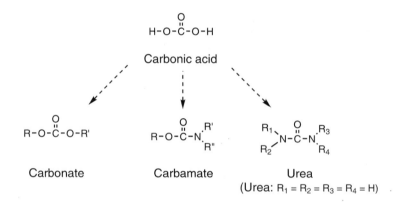

■ **NOMENCLATURE.** Carbonate nomenclature may be common or official. In either case, the two alcohol portions are named and combined with the word "carbonate" (carbonates are ester derivatives of carbonic acid). An example of carbonate nomenclature is shown in Figure 12-9.

Carbamates are ester-amide derivatives of carbonic acid and, like carbonates, require the naming of the alcohol and the amine, using either common names or IUPAC nomenclature, followed by the word "carbamate" (Fig. 12-10).

The ureas, the diamide derivatives of carbonic acid, are illustrated in Figure 12-11. In this case, it may be necessary, as we see in the example, to differentiate between the two nitrogens. This is done by using N for the one nitrogen and N' for

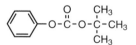

Common: Ethyl isopropyl <u>carbonate</u>   t-Butyl phenyl <u>carbonate</u>

IUPAC : Ethyl 2-Propyl <u>carbonate</u>   Phenyl 2-methyl-2-propyl <u>carbonate</u>

FIGURE 12-9. Examples of Common and Official (IUPAC) nomenclature of carbonates.

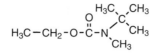

Common: Ethyl N-methyl-N-t-butyl <u>carbamate</u>

IUPAC   : Ethyl N-methyl-N-2-(2-methylpropyl) <u>carbamate</u>

FIGURE 12-10. Examples of Common and Official (IUPAC) nomenclature of carbamates.

N,N'-Diethyl-N,N'-dimethyl <u>urea</u>   N,N-Diethyl-N',N'-dimethyl <u>urea</u>

FIGURE 12-11. Examples of nomenclature of ureas.

the other nitrogen. In the preceding cases, the structures should be obvious by the use of the terms "carbonate," "carbamate," and "urea" in the nomenclature.

■ **PHYSICAL-CHEMICAL PROPERTIES.** The physical and chemical properties of the carbonate parallel those of the ester, while the properties of the urea are similar to those of the amide. The carbamate has physical properties that represent the combined effect of both components. Chemically, however, the carbamate shares reactions more like those of an ester, by which is meant that carbonates and carbamates are unstable to acid and base conditions. The ureas, being similar to amides, are relatively nonreactive solids with the polarity properties previously discussed for amides (Fig. 12-12).

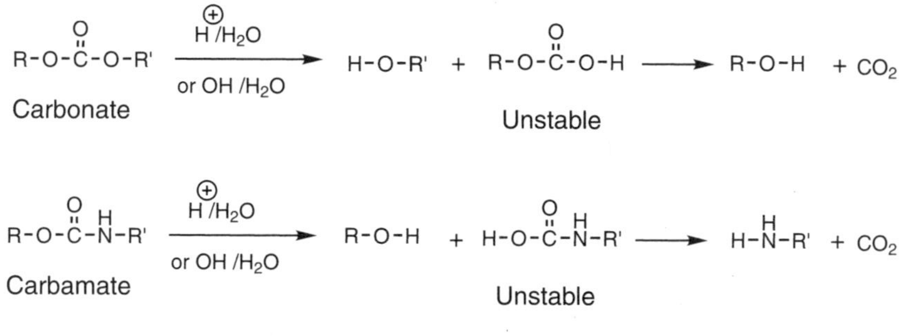

Ureas: Relatively nonreactive to aqueous acid or aqueous base

FIGURE 12-12. Acid- or base-catalyzed hydrolysis of carbonates and carbamates.

■ **METABOLISM.** The metabolic route open to these functional derivatives of carbonic acid is the hydrolysis reaction. This reaction is catalyzed by the esterase enzymes. Both the carbonate and the carbamate have the ester portion first hydrolyzed to give the monosubstituted carbonic acid. This acid is unstable and decomposes with loss of CO_2, as shown in Figure 12-13. Carbonates are hydrolyzed with formation of carbon dioxide and alcohol, and carbamates decompose to carbon dioxide, an alcohol, and an amine. The ureas are relatively stable chemicals and are not commonly metabolized by hydrolysis.

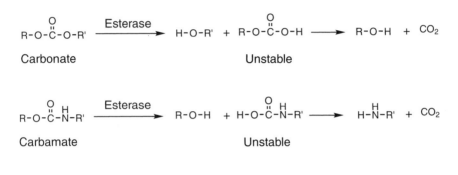

Ureas: Relatively nonreactive to esterase

FIGURE 12-13. Metabolic hydrolysis of carbonates and carbamates.

AMIDINES AND GUANIDINES

The final functional derivatives of the carboxylic acids are amidines and guanidines. Amidines are actually a functional derivative of an amide, while the guanidine is a functional derivative of urea. These two groups are mentioned since they are found as an integral part of several drug molecules. The guanidine moiety is an important unit in the naturally occurring amino acid arginine.

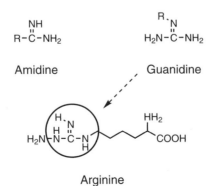

Arginine

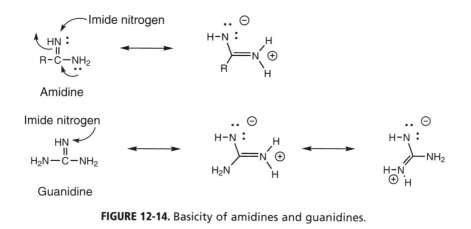

FIGURE 12-14. Basicity of amidines and guanidines.

■ **PHYSICAL-CHEMICAL PROPERTIES.** The chief characteristic of both amidines and guanidine is the high degree of basicity. In both cases the imide nitrogen maintains an unshared pair of electrons and therefore takes on a high degree of basicity. The basicity is actually increased through resonance, as indicated in Figure 12-14. The strength of this basicity is actually quite high. Amidines may have a pK_a of 9 to 10, while guanidines may have a pK_a as high as 13. The remaining nitrogen or nitrogens in the respective molecules remain neutral since, as indicated in Figure 12-14, the electron pair is shared by the nitrogen, the adjacent carbon, and to some extent the basic nitrogen.

Sulfonic Acids and Sulfonamides

13

SULFONIC ACIDS

■ **NOMENCLATURE.** A single nomenclature is used for sulfonic acids. This nomenclature is illustrated for several of the most common sulfonic acids (Fig. 13-1).

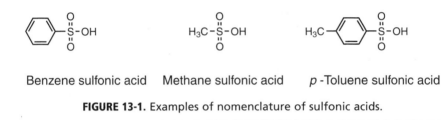

Benzene sulfonic acid   Methane sulfonic acid   *p* -Toluene sulfonic acid

FIGURE 13-1. Examples of nomenclature of sulfonic acids.

■ **PHYSICAL-CHEMICAL PROPERTIES.** A very significant physical-chemical property of the sulfonic acids is the pH characteristic. Sulfonic acids, in general, are strong acids, with pK_a's nearly as low as those of the mineral acids (Table 13-1). Saying that an acid is a strong acid implies that considerable dissociation occurs in water, and this suggests the possibility of ion-dipole interaction with water. By now one should know that such binding will favor water solubility. The solubility of several of these acids is shown in Table 13-1.

SULFONAMIDES

With this brief background, one now turns to the very important derivative of sulfonic acids, the sulfonamides. This group of compounds is important in medicinal chemistry, since a wide variety of drugs have the benzene sulfonamide nucleus.

■ **NOMENCLATURE.** The nomenclature for aryl sulfonamides is fairly straightforward. The name of the substituted benzene followed by the suffix "sulfonamide" is commonly used, although a few important common names will also have to be memorized, such as sulfanilamide (Fig. 13-2).

■ **PHYSICAL-CHEMICAL PROPERTIES.** The aryl sulfonamides tend to be solids with high melting points and poor water solubility. Similar to carboxylic acid amides, aryl

Table 13-1. WATER SOLUBILITY OF COMMON SULFONIC ACIDS

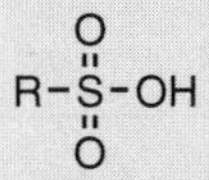 $\underset{\displaystyle O}{\overset{\displaystyle O}{R-S-OH}}$	Solubility (g/100g H_2O)	pKa in H_2O
R = H_3C—	20.0	-1.2
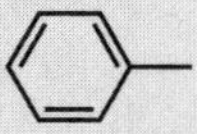 ⟨benzene⟩—	Soluble	0.7
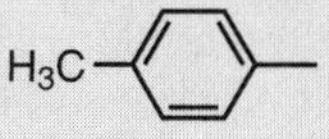 H_3C—⟨benzene⟩—	67.0	
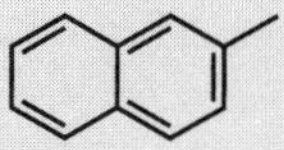 ⟨naphthalene⟩—	Soluble	

sulfonamides are chemically quite stable. Benzene sulfonamides are stable to acid, base, and enzymatic hydrolysis.

Unlike the carboxylic acid amides, which are considered neutral compounds, the aryl sulfonamides are weak acids. The acidic nature results from the ability of the SO_2 moiety to stabilize the nitrogen anion through resonance (Fig. 13-3). In the presence of a strong base, such as sodium or potassium hydroxide, aryl sul-

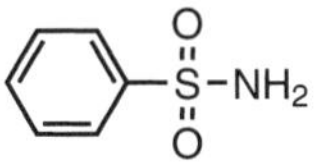

Common: Benzene sulfonamide
IUPAC:　 Benzene sulfonamide

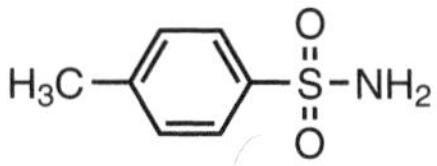

Common: *p*-Toluene sulfonamide
IUPAC: 4-Methylbenzene sulfonamide

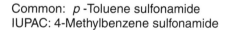

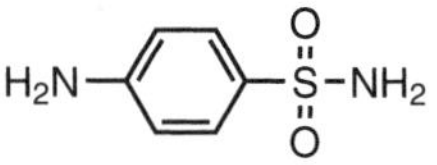

Common: *p*-Aminobenzene sulfonamide
　　　　　 Sulfanilamide
IUPAC:　　 4-Aminobenzene sulfonamide

FIGURE 13-2. Examples of nomenclature of aryl sulfonamides.

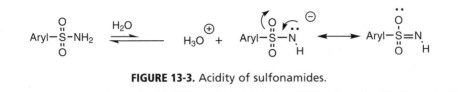

FIGURE 13-3. Acidity of sulfonamides.

fonamides will react to form a salt (Fig. 13-4). The sodium or potassium salt of a sulfonamide will readily dissociate in water, leading to highly water-soluble products, the result of ion-dipole bonding. The pH of the aqueous media following dissolution of a sodium or potassium salt of a sulfonamide tends to be quite alkaline. The water-soluble salts of aryl sulfonamides are incompatible with acidic media since an acid-base reaction can occur, usually leading to precipitation of the aryl sulfonamide.

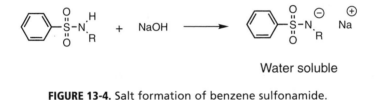

Water soluble

FIGURE 13-4. Salt formation of benzene sulfonamide.

Thioethers and Nitro Groups

14

THIOETHERS

The thioether is the sulfur analog of the previously discussed ethers. The replacement of oxygen with sulfur results in a compound with a significant increase in the boiling point and a decrease in water solubility. In general, the thioether is considered to be a lipophilic functional group. The thio ether is mentioned because it is found in a variety of drug molecules as diaryl-, dialkyl-, or arylalkylthioether (Fig. 14-1).

Of significance is the unique metabolic reaction that thio ethers may undergo. That reaction is the oxidation reaction. This may not be too surprising since sulfur exists in a variety of oxidation states, including -2, $+4$, and $+6$. The thio ether moiety may undergo a single oxidation to the sulfoxide or may be oxidized to the sulfone (Fig. 14-2).

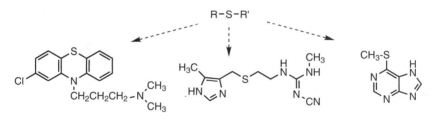

Chlorpromazine   Cimetidine   6-Methylthiopurine

FIGURE 14-1. Examples of the thioether in drug molecules.

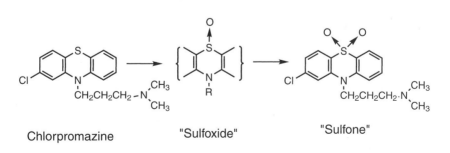

Chlorpromazine   "Sulfoxide"   "Sulfone"

FIGURE 14-2. Metabolism of thioethers.

NITRO GROUPS

The second functional group is the organic bound nitro group (Fig. 14-3). In most cases the nitro is present as an aromatic bound nitro, such as those shown in Figure 14-3. While official nomenclature may be quite complicated, one should recognize the presence of a nitro group since this group is named as "nitro" in the official nomenclature. It is also important to note that a nitro group is a charged species, as shown.

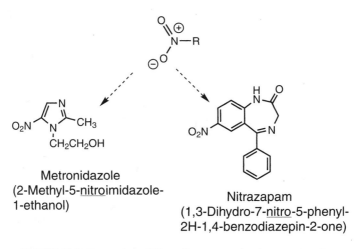

Metronidazole
(2-Methyl-5-nitroimidazole-
1-ethanol)

Nitrazapam
(1,3-Dihydro-7-nitro-5-phenyl-
2H-1,4-benzodiazepin-2-one)

FIGURE 14-3. Examples of the nitro group in drug molecules.

Metabolism of aryl nitro groups is that of reduction to the arylamine. The reduction intermediates, one of which is the hydroxylamine, have been implicated as possible carcinogens.

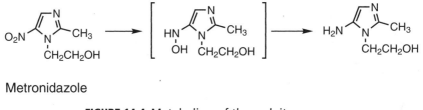

Metronidazole

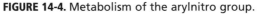

FIGURE 14-4. Metabolism of the arylnitro group.

Heterocycles

This chapter introduces the subject of heterocyclic chemistry. *Heterocycles* are defined as cyclic molecules that contain one or more heteroatoms in a ring. A *heteroatom* is an atom other than carbon. One need merely glance through an index of biologically active structures to recognize the array of heterocycles found in synthetic and naturally occurring molecules. A background in heterocyclic chemistry is therefore highly desirable. The competencies expected of you from this section of the book consist of:

1. The ability to match a structure of a heterocycle to its common or official name
2. The ability to list the physical and chemical properties of representative heterocycles
3. The ability to draw the structure of expected metabolites of common heterocycles

It would be impossible to introduce all of the possible heterocycles that are of medicinal value within the limitations of this book. I have selected a limited number of monocyclic, bicyclic, and tricyclic rings and will confine the discussion to the heteroatoms of oxygen, nitrogen, and sulfur. In addition, only three-, four-, five-, six-, seven-, and eight-membered monocyclic heterocycles will be considered, along with the five-six, six-six, and six-seven bicyclic heterocycles. Several important tricyclic rings will also be considered. In systematic nomenclature, one will recognize a consistent form of nomenclature that follows certain rules for naming the heteroatom and ring size. Tables 15-1 and 15-2 list the rules for heterocyclic systems. In addition, as will be noted in the nomenclature section for the individual heterocycles, the numbering of heterocycles usually begins with the heteroatom being designated as the 1 position. In heterocycles that contain multiple heteroatoms, the convention is that in numbering, the oxygen atom has priority over the sulfur atom, which in turn has priority over the nitrogen atom.

THREE-MEMBERED RING HETEROCYCLES

Oxygen

■ **NOMENCLATURE.** A saturated three-membered ring containing oxygen is known as the oxirane (Fig. 15-1) ring according to the rules presented in Tables 15-1 and 15-2. While correctly named as oxiranes, the common practice for such mol-

Table 15-1. ACCEPTABLE PREFIXES FOR COMMON HETEROATOMS

Element	Prefix
Oxygen	Oxa
Nitrogen	Aza
Sulfur	Thia

Table 15-2. COMMON SUFFIXES FOR NITROGEN-CONTAINING HETEROCYCLES AND NON-NITROGEN-CONTAINING HETEROCYCLES BASED ON RING SIZE

Ring Size	Saturated	Partly Saturated	Unsaturated
	Rings With Nitrogen		
3	-iridine		-irine
5	-olidine	-oline	-ole
6	-ine	(di or tetrahydro)	-ine
7	(hexahydro)	(di or tetrahydro)	-epine
8	(octahydro)	(di, tetra, or hexahydro)	-ocine
	Rings Without Nitrogen		
3	-irane		-irene
5	-olane	-olene	-ole
6	-ane	(di or tetrahydro)	-ine
7	-epane	(di or tetrahydro)	-epine
8	-ocane	(di, tetra, or hexahydro)	-ocin

ecules is to refer to these agents as epoxides. A number of natural products can be found that contain the epoxide functional group, and you will be introduced to additional epoxide-containing drugs in medicinal chemistry.

■ **PHYSICAL-CHEMICAL PROPERTIES.** Epoxides are ethers, but because of the three-membered ring, epoxides have unusual properties. The three-membered ring forces the atoms making up the ring to have an average bond angle of 60°, considerably less than the normal tetrahedral bond angle of 109.5°. This highly

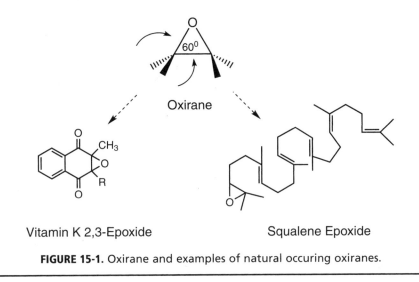

Vitamin K 2,3-Epoxide   Squalene Epoxide

FIGURE 15-1. Oxirane and examples of natural occuring oxiranes.

strained ring therefore readily opens in the presence of either acid or base cata-
lysts, as shown in Figure 15-2. These reactions are important, since drugs that contain an epoxide ring are also quite reactive both in vitro and in vivo. Such drugs will
react with a nucleophile (N:) in the presence of acid or will react with a base that
acts as a nucleophile to give open-chain compounds. When drugs containing epoxides are administered to a patient, the epoxide can be expected to react with
biopolymers (e.g., proteins), leading to destructive effects on the cell. Such drugs
may find use in cancer chemotherapy but are usually found to be quite toxic.

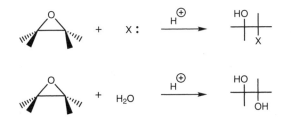

FIGURE 15-2. Acid- or base-catalyzed ring opening reactions of epoxides.

Nitrogen

■ **NOMENCLATURE.** A saturated three-membered ring containing nitrogen is
known as the aziridine ring (Fig. 15-3). This is the only nomenclature used for such
a unit. Although aziridine rings are not common in nature or in many drugs, their
intermediacy is required and accounts for the biologic activity of a specific class of
anticancer drugs known as the nitrogen mustards.

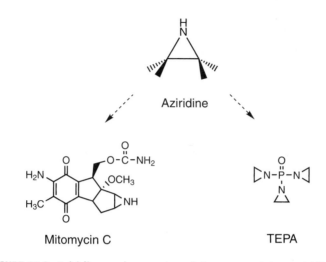

FIGURE 15-3. Aziridine and examples of drugs containing aziridines.

■ **PHYSICAL-CHEMICAL PROPERTIES.** Similar to the properties of the epoxide, aziridines are highly strained, highly reactive molecules. The anticancer drug mechlorethamine (Fig. 15-4) owes its activity to the formation of a charged intermediate aziridine (aziridinium ion). Because of its high reactivity, aziridine will react with most nucleophiles (N:), including water. If the nucleophile is part of a biopolymer, this reaction, known as an alkylation reaction, can result in the death of the cell. This reaction is either beneficial, where the cell is a cancer cell, or the mechanism of toxicity, where the cell is a host cell. The drug mechlorethamine has only a short half-life when dissolved in water because the aziridinium ion, when formed, reacts with water to give an alcohol that does not possess biologic activity.

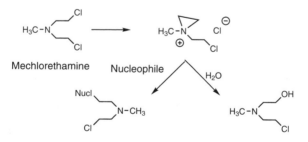

FIGURE 15-4. Aziridine as a reactive intermediate formed from mechlorethamine.

FOUR-MEMBERED RING HETEROCYCLES

Only one derivative of a four-membered ring heterocycle will be mentioned here. This system is the β-lactam, a unit found in the penicillin and cephalosporin antibi-

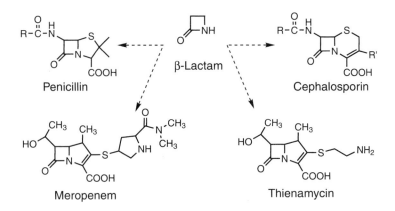

FIGURE 15-5. β-Lactam and examples of drugs containing the β-lactam.

otics as well as a number of derivatives, both synthetic and naturally occurring, of these well-known antibiotics (Fig. 15-5). The nomenclature for this heterocycle is derived from the fact that cyclic amides are known as lactams, and this particular system results from cyclization of a β-aminocarboxylic acid, thus the β-lactam name. The notable property of the β-lactam, its ease of hydrolysis by aqueous acid, aqueous base, and enzymatic conditions, results from the considerable strain energy found in this molecule. The four-membered ring distorts the normal bond angles for carbon, but additionally the presence of the sp^2 carbonyl carbon adds to this strain. The hydrolysis of the β-lactam (Fig. 15-6) is a significant problem experienced by many of the penicillins, cephalosporins, and other β-lactam-containing antibiotics.

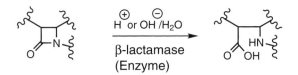

FIGURE 15-6. Hydrolysis of β-lactams.

FIVE-MEMBERED RING HETEROCYCLES

Oxygen

■ **NOMENCLATURE.** Two common five-membered ring heterocycles are furan and tetrahydrofuran (Fig. 15-7). With this ring system, you need not be concerned with official nomenclature; the common or trivial name will be used in nearly all cases. Substituted furans and tetrahydrofurans are numbered starting with the

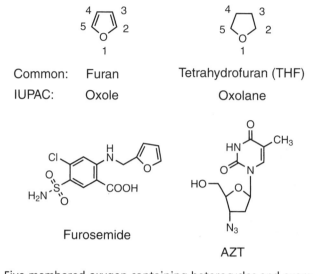

Common: Furan   Tetrahydrofuran (THF)

IUPAC: Oxole   Oxolane

Furosemide

AZT

FIGURE 15-7. Five-membered oxygen containing heterocycles and examples of drugs containing these rings.

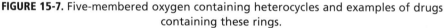

oxygen as the 1 position and numbering the ring such that any substituents receive the next lowest number.

A number of furan-containing drugs can be found, while virtually no pure tetrahydrofuran-containing drugs exist. What appears to be a tetrahydrofuran is seen in the ribose-containing anticancer and antiviral drugs, but these sugars are actually mixed acetal structures.

■ **PHYSICAL-CHEMICAL PROPERTIES.** Although furan looks like an ether, it does not behave like one; its properties are more like those of benzene. Furan is an aromatic ring. You may recall that aromatic rings are flat molecules that contain $4N + 2\pi$ electrons, in which $N = 1, 2, 3$, etc. If one considers the π electrons or sp^2 electrons present in furan, it will be noted that furan contains four π electrons in the two double bonds and two pairs of sp^2 electrons on the oxygen. One pair of the electrons on oxygen is in the same plane with the four π electrons of the two double bonds, thus resulting in a cloud of six electrons located above and below the plane of the ring (Fig. 15-8). Furan therefore has the properties of an aromatic compound: namely, it is relatively nonreactive under the conditions encountered in pharmacy. On the other hand, tetrahydrofuran has quite different properties when compared to furan. Tetrahydrofuran is simply a cyclic ether but unlike its closest open-chain relative, diethylether, does not show partial water solubility; it is highly soluble in water. This is due to the strong bonding between the hydrogen of water and the unshared pairs of electrons on the ether oxygen (Fig. 15-9).

Tetrahydrofuran is easily oxidized in the presence of air to give peroxides and, like most ethers, also must be protected from atmospheric oxygen.

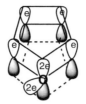

FIGURE 15-8. π electron structure of furan.

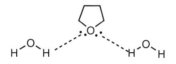

FIGURE 15-9. Strong dipole-dipole bonding in THF leading to increased water solubility.

■ **METABOLISM.** The metabolism of furan and tetrahydrofuran follow the pattern expected for an aromatic compound and an ether, respectively. While tetrahydrofuran is relatively stable in vivo, furan may undergo the expected aromatic hydroxylation (Fig. 15-10).

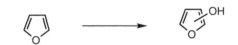

FIGURE 15-10. Metabolic hydroxylation of furan.

Nitrogen

■ **NOMENCLATURE.** Two common five-membered ring heterocycles containing nitrogen are pyrrole and pyrrolidine (Fig. 15-11). Here again, the common name should be learned; the official name can be neglected since it is seldom used. For substituted pyrroles or pyrrolidines, the numbering starts with nitrogen and proceeds clockwise or counterclockwise to give any substituent present the next lowest number. The pyrrole and pyrrolidine heterocycles are common features in many drugs and naturally occurring substances.

■ **PHYSICAL-CHEMICAL PROPERTIES.** Pyrrole, like furan, is an aromatic compound. It is an aromatic compound that is a weak base and, for our purposes, will be considered neutral. This property can be explained by accounting for all of the nonbonding electrons present in pyrrole (Fig. 15-12). Nitrogen's extra pair of electrons, which are usually available for sharing and account for the basic properties of

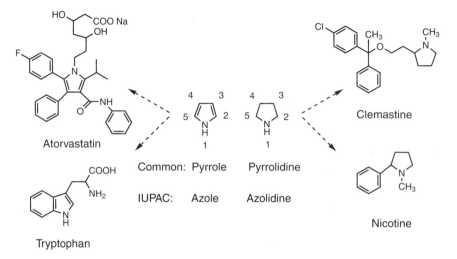

FIGURE 15-11. Pyrrole and pyrrolidine and examples of drugs containing these heterocycles.

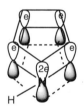

FIGURE 15-12. π electron structure of pyrrole.

amines, are not available for sharing. This pair of electrons is part of the π cloud of electrons.

In the fully reduced heterocycle, pyrrolidine, one is dealing with a secondary amine with properties equivalent to any other secondary amine. Unlike pyrrole, with a pK_a of the protonated pyrrole of approximately 0.4, pyrrolidine is a strong base, with a pK_a of the ammonium ion of approximately 11. As might be expected, pyrrolidine, with only four carbon atoms and the availability of an unshared pair of electrons for hydrogen bonding, is quite water-soluble.

■ **METABOLISM.** The metabolism of pyrrole and pyrrolidine, as well as of pyrrole- and pyrrolidine-containing molecules, follows the pattern expected for an aromatic compound and a secondary amine, respectively. Aromatic hydroxylation would be predicted for pyrrole, while pyrrolidine could be expected to undergo conjugation with glucuronic acid or sulfuric acid. Acetylation, a common reaction for secondary amines, might also be expected to occur (see Fig. 10-10, page 46)

Sulfur

■ **NOMENCLATURE.** As with the previous oxygen and nitrogen heterocycles, two sulfur-containing heterocycles, thiophene and tetrahydrothiophene, exist. Here again, the common nomenclature is used in most instances. With substituted analogs, the numbering of the rings starts with the heteroatom, proceeding either clockwise or counterclockwise, such that any substituent receives the next lowest number (Fig. 15-13). While the thiophene nucleus is common in drug molecules, the tetrahydrothiophene is quite uncommon.

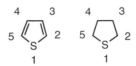

Common: Thiophene Tetrahydrothiophene

IUPAC: Thiole   Thiolane

Sufentanil   Methapyrilene

FIGURE 15-13. Thiophene and tetrahydrothiophene and examples of drugs containing the thiophene heterocycle.

■ **PHYSICAL-CHEMICAL PROPERTIES.** The properties of the five-membered sulfur-containing heterocycles are based upon the proper recognition of the class of compounds to which they belong. Thiophene is an aromatic ring and is therefore relatively stable, while tetrahydrothiophene is a thioether. Unlike oxygen ethers, the thioethers are fairly stable compounds and, also unlike the oxygen analogs, the sulfur-containing compounds are less water-soluble. In general, the substitution of sulfur for oxygen results in a significant decrease in hydrophilic character and a corresponding increase in lipophilic character.

■ **METABOLISM.** The predicted metabolic pattern for thiophene is aromatic hydroxylation, with hydroxylation occurring at any hydrogen-substituted position. For reduced thiophenes, tetrahydrothiophene, oxidation of sulfur would be pre-

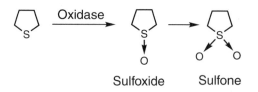

Sulfoxide   Sulfone

FIGURE 15-14. Metabolic oxidation of tetrahydrothiophene.

dicted to occur. This was previously discussed for thioethers and is again shown in Figure 15-14.

FIVE-MEMBERED RING HETEROCYCLES WITH TWO OR MORE HETEROATOMS

Oxygen and Nitrogen

■ **NOMENCLATURE.** Oxygen-plus-nitrogen in a five-membered ring gives rise to the heterocycles oxazole and isoxazole. The oxazole nomenclature is similar to its official name, but for convenience the -1,3- is dropped, and it is understood that oxazole consists of the 1,3 arrangement of oxygen and nitrogen. The only other arrangement of these two atoms in a five-membered ring would be the 1,2 placement. Since this is an isomer of oxazole, the common name is isoxazole (Fig. 15-15). As indicated previously, the numbering of the ring proceeds from oxygen at the 1 position to nitrogen such that the nitrogen is the next lowest position (i.e., 3 in oxazole or 2 in isoxazole).

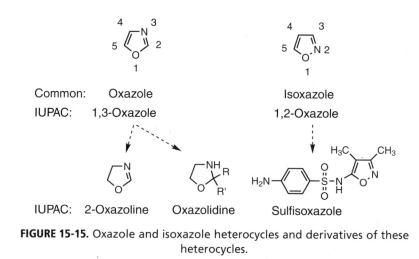

FIGURE 15-15. Oxazole and isoxazole heterocycles and derivatives of these heterocycles.

The partially and totally reduced derivatives of oxazole are also shown. The nomenclature is based upon the general rules presented in Table 15-2. Depending on the substitution at the two position, oxazolidine is actually a mixed acetal (R = H, alkyl or aryl; R' = H) or a mixed ketal (R = alkyl, aryl; R' = alkyl or aryl) (see page 36)

▪ **PHYSICAL-CHEMICAL PROPERTIES.** Both oxazole and isoxazole are aromatic compounds. The aromatic π cloud is made up of two electrons from each double bond, plus a pair of electrons contributed by the oxygen atom. Since nitrogen is left with its unshared pair of electrons, both of these compounds are basic, although they should be recognized as weak bases ($pK_a < 6.0$ of the protonated nitrogen) (Fig. 15-16). Both compounds can be converted to salts with a strong acid such as hydrochloric acid. As their hydrochloric salts, oxazoles and isoxazoles would be predicted to be water-soluble.

2-Oxazoline and oxazolidine are also basic compounds but prove unstable in aqueous acid media. An example of such instability is shown in Figure 15-17.

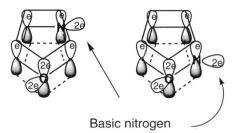

Basic nitrogen

FIGURE 15-16. π electron structure of oxazole and isoxazole.

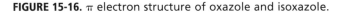

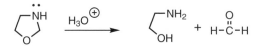

FIGURE 15-17. Acid catalyzed hydrolysis of oxazolidine.

▪ **METABOLISM.** The only characteristic metabolism of significance is aromatic hydroxylation. In the case of oxazole, the product formed exists in the "keto" form shown in Figure 15-18.

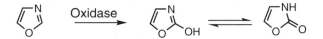

Figure 15-18. Metabolic hydroxylation of oxazole.

Nitrogen and Nitrogen

■ **NOMENCLATURE.** Two important dinitrogen heterocycles are found in medicinal agents; these are imidazole and pyrazole (Fig. 15-19). As with several previous examples, the student should be familiar with the common name, since it is used in most cases. The important partially reduced and saturated analogs of imidazole are 2-imidazoline and imidazolidine, respectively. These compounds are numbered similarly to that shown for imidazole.

There are a variety of imidazole-containing drugs but far fewer pyrazole-containing agents.

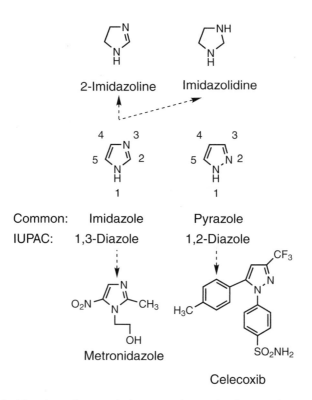

FIGURE 15-19. Imidazole and pyrazole heterocycles, reduction products of imidazole, and derivatives of imidazole and pyrazole.

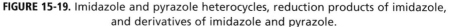

■ **PHYSICAL-CHEMICAL PROPERTIES.** Pyrazole and imidazole are both aromatic compounds that have one basic nitrogen and a neutral nitrogen. The aromatic nature arises from the four π electrons and the unshared pair of electrons on the -NH- nitrogen. Some care should be taken in specifying which nitrogen is basic since, in unsymmetrical derivatives, resonance prevents one from isolating a specific compound, as shown in Figure 15-20. All that can be said is that one nitrogen is basic.

In 2-imidazoline, both nitrogens are basic. The 2° amine is more basic than the sp² nitrogen, but again it may not be possible to specify which is sp³ and which is sp². Imidazolidine, on the other hand, is made up of two 2° amines and is quite basic. Imidazolidine, like oxazolidine, is unstable in aqueous acid and is hydrolyzed to ethylenediamine and formaldehyde (Fig. 15-21). This again is related to the fact that imidazolidine is an acetal derivative.

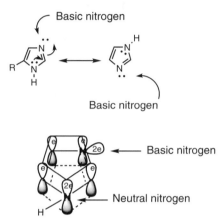

FIGURE 15-20. The imidazole heterocycle has one basic nitrogen, which, because of resonance, may be either nitrogen.

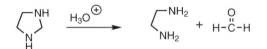

FIGURE 15-21. Acid catalyzed hydrolysis of imidazolidine.

■ **METABOLISM.** The predicted metabolism is uneventful. While the aromatic compounds may be prone to hydroxylation, the reduced heterocycles would be expected to act like secondary amines in vivo and undergo conjugation reactions.

Nitrogen and Sulfur

■ **NOMENCLATURE.** The only heterocycle to be considered that contains a nitrogen and sulfur in a five-membered ring is the chemical 1,3-thiazole (Fig. 15-22). The nomenclature used is that derived from Tables 15-1 and 15-2. The thiazole nucleus is a very common moiety found in many drug molecules.

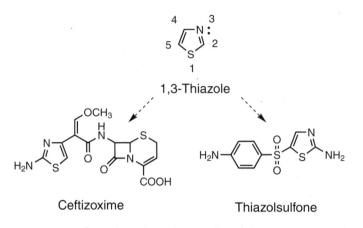

Ceftizoxime   **Thiazolsulfone**

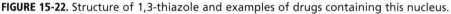

FIGURE 15-22. Structure of 1,3-thiazole and examples of drugs containing this nucleus.

■ **PHYSICAL-CHEMICAL PROPERTIES.** The properties of thiazole are similar to those of oxazole. This compound is aromatic, and the nitrogen in this compound with its unshared pair of electrons is basic.

■ **METABOLISM.** The metabolic properties are analogous to those of the other aromatic heterocycles and consist of aromatic hydroxylation at any of the carbon hydrogen locations.

Complex Five-Membered Heterocycles

■ **NOMENCLATURE.** A series of miscellaneous heterocycles important to medicinal chemistry are shown in this section, along with a few examples of drugs containing these heterocycles. The 1,3,4-thiadiazole and 1,2,5-thiadiazole have nomenclature that is self-explanatory and follows the priority rules previously mentioned and the abbreviations for the heteroatoms (a sulfur, two nitrogens in a five-membered ring) (Fig. 15-23).

Several triazoles exist, in which the "tri" indicates three, "az" signifies nitrogen, and "ole" indicates a five-membered ring (Fig. 15-24). If the three nitrogens are symmetrically arranged (at the 1, 3, and 4 positions), the compound can be identified as s-Triazole ("s" for symmetrical), while if not symmetrically arranged the compound is named 1H-1,2,4-triazole. One additional poly nitrogen-containing heterocycle is tetrazole.

The oxazolidinone and oxazolidindione nomenclature should be understandable based on the oxazolidine nomenclature explained earlier, with the "one" signifying a carbonyl and "dione" representing two carbonyls at the 2 and 4 positions (Fig. 15-25).

One additional important heterocycle is the hydantoin nucleus. Here the common nomenclature replaces the official nomenclature of imidazolidindione. A number of very important classes of drugs possess these heterocyclic nuclei.

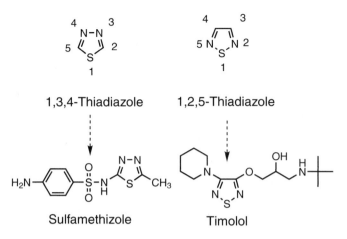

1,3,4-Thiadiazole   1,2,5-Thiadiazole

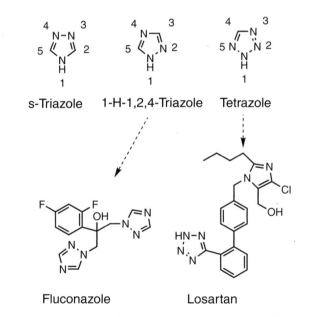

Sulfamethizole   Timolol

FIGURE 15-23. Structure of thiadiazoles and examples of drugs containing this nucleus.

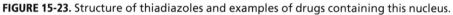

s-Triazole   1-H-1,2,4-Triazole   Tetrazole

Fluconazole   Losartan

FIGURE 15-24. Structure of triazoles, tetrazole and examples of drugs containing these nuclei.

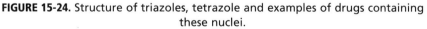

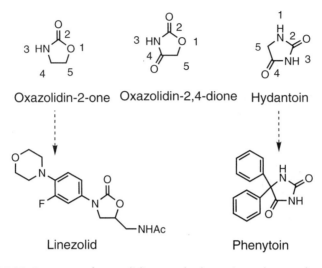

Oxazolidin-2-one   Oxazolidin-2,4-dione   Hydantoin

Linezolid   Phenytoin

FIGURE 15-25. Structure of oxazolidinones, hydrantoin and examples of drugs containing these nuclei.

■ **PHYSICAL-CHEMICAL PROPERTIES.** The thiadiazoles, triazoles, and tetrazoles are typical aromatic nuclei that have two (thiadiazole, triazole) or three (tetrazole) basic nitrogens in the ring. If one accounts for the electrons required for aromaticity, it should be obvious which nitrogens retain the electrons necessary for basicity. Little additional information is necessary, since none of these compounds has any unique physical-chemical properties that one needs to be concerned with.

The oxazolidin-2-ones are cyclic analogs of a class of compounds discussed previously, namely the carbamates. Like their straight-chain relatives, the oxazolidin-2-ones are readily hydrolyzed by acid or basic media (Fig. 15-26).

The oxazolidin-2,4-diones do have a chemical property unique to the "imide" portion of the structure (Fig. 15-27). Although an amide is neutral, the addition of a second carbonyl covalently bonded to the nitrogen produces the imide functional group, which has acidic properties. Two electron-withdrawing groups on either side of the -NH- group withdraw the unshared pair of electrons on the nitrogen as well as the electron pair remaining after dissociation of the hydrogen. This allows the hydrogen to be abstracted by a strong base, forming an alkaline salt that is quite water-soluble.

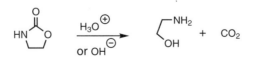

FIGURE 15-26. Acid- or base-catalyzed hydrolysis of oxazolidin-2-one.

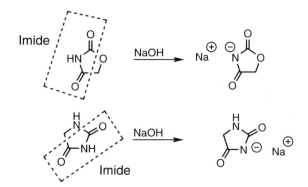

FIGURE 15-27. Salt formation at the imide nitrogen of oxazolidin-2,4-dione and hydantoin.

The final heterocycle, the hydantoin, is a cyclic urea, but in addition it contains an imide functional group. The presence of the hydrogen on the imide nitrogen again results in a compound with acidic properties.

SIX-MEMBERED RING HETEROCYCLES

Nitrogen

■ **NOMENCLATURE.** The important six-membered ring nitrogen-containing heterocycles are pyridine, the aromatic compound, and piperidine, the saturated compound (Fig. 15-28). While both common and IUPAC nomenclature is shown, in

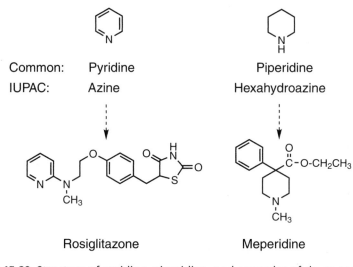

FIGURE 15-28. Structure of pyridine, piperidine, and examples of drugs containing these nuclei.

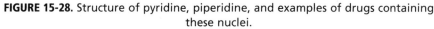

most cases the common name is used exclusively. These two heterocycles are commonly found in a variety of medicinal agents.

■ **PHYSICAL-CHEMICAL PROPERTIES.** Pyridine, unlike its carbon analog benzene, is quite water-soluble. The explanation for this fact lies in the availability of an unshared pair of electrons found on the nitrogen. This polar compound can hydrogen bond to water through this pair of electrons. The availability of the electrons accounts for the other property of pyridine that makes it different from pyrrole, namely the basicity of pyridine. Pyridinium ion has a pK_a of 5.36, which can be compared with the nearly neutral pyrrole's pK_a of 0.398, yet pyridine is much less basic than alkylamines, which have pK_a's of approximately 10 for the alkylammonium ions. Pyridine and substituted pyridines have approximately the same basicity as the aromatic ammonium ions such as aniline (pK_a of 4.6). Thus, it would be difficult to predict a difference in basicity between the two nitrogens in the following compound:

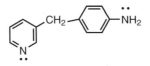

On the other hand, piperidine is nothing more than a cyclic alkyl amine. It is quite basic, with a $pK_a \approx 11.3$ for the piperidinium ion. Other than the reactivity of pyridine and piperidine toward strong acids, one should consider both of these compounds as relatively stable.

■ **METABOLISM.** Pyridine, since it is an aromatic compound, acts like the typical aromatic rings and undergoes hydroxylation. Piperidine acts like a typical secondary amine and would be predicted to undergo conjugation with glucuronic acid or sulfuric acid.

Dealkylation resulting in ring cleavage would not be expected to occur with piperidine, since dealkylation occurs primarily with amines that are substituted with smaller alkyl groups such as methyl or ethyl groups.

SIX-MEMBERED RING HETEROCYCLES WITH TWO HETEROATOMS

Nitrogen and Nitrogen

■ **NOMENCLATURE.** Several important heterocycles are formed from two nitrogens in a six-membered ring, and these are shown here with their respective nomenclature (Fig. 15-29). Once again, the official nomenclature is usually neglected in favor of common nomenclature.

■ **PHYSICAL-CHEMICAL PROPERTIES.** All three of the compounds shown in Figure 15-29 have properties similar to each other and similar to the properties of pyridine. The compounds are basic and of the same order of basicity as pyridine. Since

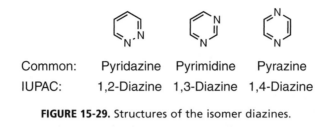

Common:	Pyridazine	Pyrimidine	Pyrazine
IUPAC:	1,2-Diazine	1,3-Diazine	1,4-Diazine

FIGURE 15-29. Structures of the isomer diazines.

these compounds are aromatic, they are also expected to be relatively nonreactive. Finally, parallel to the solubility properties of pyridine, these compounds are also water-soluble.

Pyrimidines—I

■ **NOMENCLATURE.** Three pyrimidine derivatives that are important to the structure of DNA and RNA, as well as to the structure of medicinally active agents, are shown in Figure 15-30. While official nomenclature can be derived for these compounds, it is replaced with the common names presented. Thymine may also be

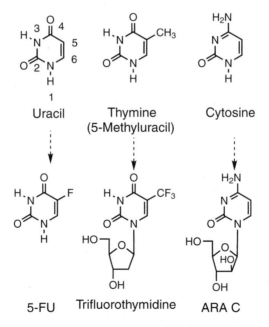

FIGURE 15-30. Structures of functionalized pyrimidines and examples of drugs containing these nuclei.

referred to as 5-methyluracil. It is important to recognize the numbering system of these heterocycles. A clockwise direction is chosen such that the heteroatoms appear at the 1 and 3 positions and the carbonyls or carbonyl and amine are at the 2 and 4 positions, respectively. If the numbering were counterclockwise, the substituents on the ring would be at the 2 and 6 positions. The pyrimidine nucleus is especially important in anticancer and antiviral drugs.

■ **PHYSICAL-CHEMICAL PROPERTIES.** The substituted pyrimidines are complex molecules because of the nature of the substituents. Uracil and thymine may be considered to contain the neutral urea unit or the acidic imide moiety, as shown in Figure 15-31, but they can also be considered to exist in either the "keto" form or "enol" form, as shown in Figure 15-32. The "enol" form would be expected to have the acidic properties of a diphenolic compound and the basic properties of a pyrimidine. Since the compounds prefer the "keto" form, they are usually thought of as weak acids, but the weak acid-weak base properties of the "enol" form may account for the reduced solubility in water of uracil and thymine. Cytosine, with the 4-amino substituent and without an imide moiety, might be expected to be a weak base.

None of the substituted pyrimidines has any noteworthy instabilities.

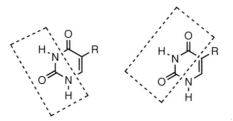

FIGURE 15-31. Structural units of the uracil nucleus.

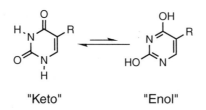

"Keto"   "Enol"

FIGURE 15-32. "Keto"-"enol" equalibrium of the uracil ring.

■ **METABOLISM.** The metabolism of these unique pyrimidines is important from the standpoint of both biochemical utilization of these compounds and drug metabolism of pyrimidine derivatives. Figure 15-33 outlines a pathway that converts uracil to a useful compound, uridylic acid, needed for the synthesis of RNA.

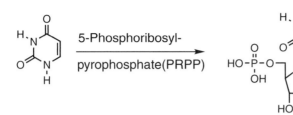

Uridine-5'-pyrophosphate
(Uridylic acid)

FIGURE 15-33. Metabolism of uracil.

In a similar manner to that shown for uracil, cytosine is conjugated with PRPP to yield cytidine-5'-monophosphate (CMP) or cytidylic acid. Thymine is metabolized by conjugation, via a salvage pathway, with PRPP to the thymine ribosyl-5'-phosphate. This form of thymidylic acid can be utilized in specific RNA molecules. The biochemically important thymine deoxyribosyl-5'-phosphate is important in the biosynthesis of DNA but is derived from uridylic acid, which is first converted to deoxyuridylic acid and then into the deoxythymidylic acid (Fig. 15-34).

An example of a pyrimidine-substituted drug and its metabolic pattern is shown in Figure 15-35. 5-Fluorouracil can be conjugated with either ribose or deoxyribose, and the sugar is then phosphorylated to either 5-fluorouridine monophosphate (5-FUMP) or 5-fluorouridine-2'-deoxyribosyl phosphate (5-FUDR). In this particular example, the 5-FUMP is responsible for the side effects of the drug, while 5-FUDR is responsible for the chemotherapeutic action of 5-FU. 5-FU is an example of an administered drug that must be "activated"; that is, it must be converted to an active drug to produce its intended pharmacologic action. Drugs such as 5-FU are referred to as "pro-drugs" since they come before the actual "active" drug (5-FUDR).

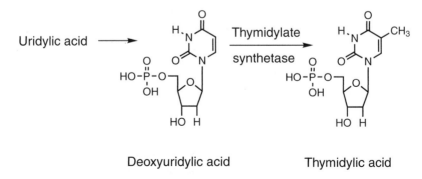

Deoxyuridylic acid   Thymidylic acid

FIGURE 15-34. Biosynthesis of thymidylic acid.

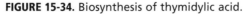

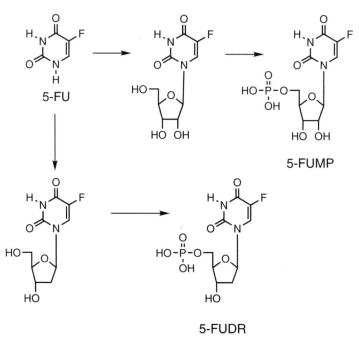

FIGURE 15-35. Metabolism of 5-fluorouracil.

Pyrimidines—II

■ **NOMENCLATURE.** Two additional special pyrimidines are barbituric acid and the substituted barbiturates (Fig. 15-36). The substituted barbiturates represent a special class of compounds that have been used for their sedative-hypnotic action since the early 1900s. The numbering system starts with either nitrogen and proceeds such that the substituents (R) appear at the 5 position.

■ **PHYSICAL-CHEMICAL PROPERTIES.** Barbituric acid can exist in any of the four forms shown in Figure 15-37. Roentgenographic studies have shown that as a solid, the compound exists in the trioxo form, while in solution evidence rules against the trihydroxy form but supports the presence of the other enolic forms.

Barbituric acid is a fairly strong acid with a pKa of 4.12, but upon substitution at the 5 position, the pKa rises dramatically. The 5,5-disubstituted barbiturates have pKa values of 7.1 to 8.1. Such compounds exist predominantly in the trioxo tautomeric form (Fig. 15-38). The 5,5-disubstituted barbiturates react with sodium hydroxide to form a salt that is quite water-soluble (Fig. 15-39). Such salts, when added to water, result in an aqueous medium that becomes quite alkaline owing to the fact that such a salt is made up of a weak acid and a strong base. If the pH of the medium is titrated to a neutral or acidic pH, the reaction will be reversed, resulting in precipitation of barbituric acid.

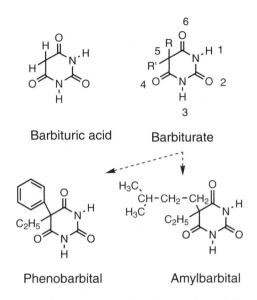

Barbituric acid   Barbiturate

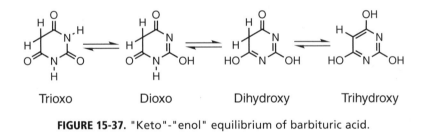

Phenobarbital   Amylbarbital

FIGURE 15-36. Structure of barbituric acid and examples of drugs containing the barbiturate nucleus.

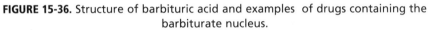

Trioxo   Dioxo   Dihydroxy   Trihydroxy

FIGURE 15-37. "Keto"-"enol" equilibrium of barbituric acid.

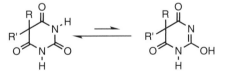

FIGURE 15-38. "Keto"-"enol" equilibrium of 5,5-disubstituted barbituric acids.

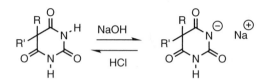

FIGURE 15-39. Salt formation of 5,5-disubstituted barbituric acids.

SATURATED SIX-MEMBERED HETEROCYCLES

■ **NOMENCLATURE.** Two important saturated heterocycles that appear in drug molecules are piperazine and morpholine (Fig. 15-40). The common names are used in nearly all cases when referring to these nuclei.

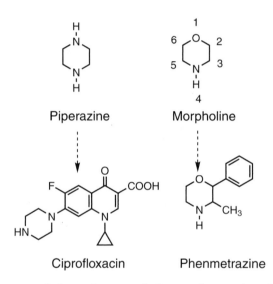

FIGURE 15-40. Structure of piperazine, morpholine, and examples of drugs containing these nuclei.

■ **PHYSICAL-CHEMICAL PROPERTIES.** Since these compounds are cyclic forms of a diamine, piperazine, and a secondary amine plus an ether, morpholine, the properties are the same as those reviewed in the chapters on these respective functional groups and need not be discussed at this point.

SEVEN- AND EIGHT-MEMBERED RING HETEROCYCLES

Nitrogen

■ **NOMENCLATURE.** Two heterocycles that complete our review of monocyclic heterocycles are hexahydroazepine and octahydroazocine (Fig. 15-41). The fully

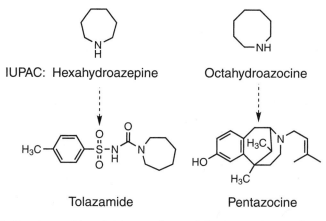

IUPAC: Hexahydroazepine   Octahydroazocine

Tolazamide   Pentazocine

FIGURE 15-41. Structure of hexahydroazepine, octahydroazocine, and an example of a drug containing the hydroazocine nucleus.

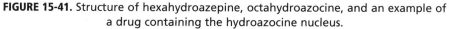

reduced azepine and azocine appear in a number of medicinal agents, and in addition the azepine is part of a tricyclic ring system that will be discussed later in the chapter.

▪ **PHYSICAL-CHEMICAL PROPERTIES.**   Both hexahydroazepine and octahydroazocine are cyclic secondary amines that are basic compounds and act like ordinary alkylamines.

BICYCLIC HETEROCYCLES: FIVE-MEMBERED RING PLUS SIX-MEMBERED RING

One Nitrogen

▪ **NOMENCLATURE.** An important bicyclic ring system containing a single nitrogen is indole. This nucleus is present in the amino acid tryptophan and is found in many alkaloids. Less important from a medicinal standpoint is the isomer of indole, isoindole (Fig. 15-42).

▪ **PHYSICAL-CHEMICAL PROPERTIES.** Indole is an aromatic compound with delocalization of the electrons across both rings (Fig. 15-43). Thus, like pyrrole, the benzopyrroles require the unshared pair of electrons on nitrogen to participate in the delocalized cloud of electrons. The result of this delocalization is that indole is a weak base and for our purposes will be considered neutral.

Indole and drugs containing the indole nucleus are easily oxidized when allowed to stand in contact with air. An indication of this reaction is the darkening of the color of the compound. It is best if indole-containing drugs are protected from atmospheric oxygen by storing under nitrogen.

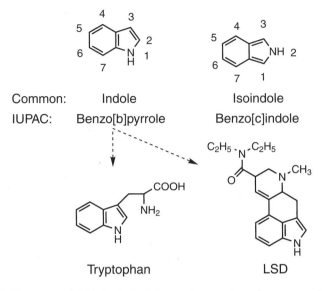

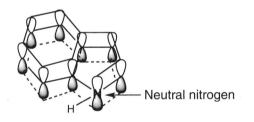

FIGURE 15-42. Structure of indole, isoindole, and examples of compounds containing these nuclei.

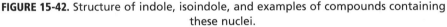

FIGURE 15-43. π electron structure of indole.

■ **METABOLISM.** Since indole is an aromatic nucleus, it is expected that aromatic hydroxylation would occur. Most indole-containing drugs are substituted at the 3 position, and the hydroxylation occurs at the 4–7 position of the molecule.

Two Heteroatoms

■ **NOMENCLATURE.** Three bicyclic heterocycles that contain two heteroatoms are shown in Figure 15-44. The common nomenclature is based upon the name of the five-membered ring, and since it is fused to a benzene ring, they are referred to as benz(o) ("o" is dropped when followed by a vowel) and then the name of the five-membered ring heterocycle. The numbering proceeds as shown. The bridgehead positions (e.g., the positions where the two rings join) are not numbered because

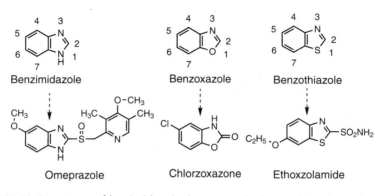

FIGURE 15-44. Structures of benimidazole, benzoxazole, benzothiazole, and examples of drugs containing these nuclei.

the carbons at the bridgehead are already fully substituted. In cases in which the benzene ring is reduced, the bridgehead position can be numbered at the 3a and 7a positions since they follow the 3 and 7 positions, respectively.

■ **PHYSICAL-CHEMICAL PROPERTIES.** The properties of the benzimidazole, benzoxazole, and benzothiazole do not differ significantly from the properties of imidazole, oxazole, or thiazole. All three compounds are aromatic, and all three have a weakly basic nitrogen in the molecule. The only property that does change is the fact that the molecules are less water-soluble, since each has four additional carbon atoms present.

■ **METABOLISM.** The predicted metabolism of these heterocycles is aromatic hydroxylation. The hydroxylation can occur at any of the positions occupied by hydrogen (2, 4, 5, 6, or 7 positions).

Four Heteroatoms

■ **NOMENCLATURE.** An important bicyclic heterocycle is the purine nucleus (Fig. 15-45). The purine can be thought of as a pyrimidine fused to an imidazole. The numbering follows this type of analogy. The six-membered ring is numbered first, starting with one nitrogen atom and proceeding counterclockwise completely around the ring, including the bridgehead positions. This is then followed by numbering the five-membered ring.

Three common substituted purines should be familiar to the reader and are also shown in Figure 15-45. They include the 6-aminopurine (adenine), 2-amino-6-hydroxypurine (guanine) (which actually exists not in the "enol" but rather in the "keto" form), and 2,6-purinedione (xanthine). All three of these compounds are common metabolites found in the human body and are important nuclei in a number of drug molecules.

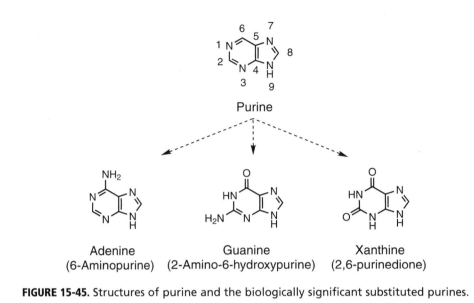

Purine

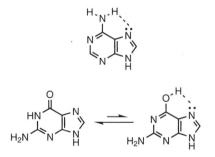

Adenine   Guanine   Xanthine
(6-Aminopurine)   (2-Amino-6-hydroxypurine)   (2,6-purinedione)

FIGURE 15-45. Structures of purine and the biologically significant substituted purines.

■ **PHYSICAL-CHEMICAL PROPERTIES.** Purine is an aromatic compound containing three basic nitrogens. Because of the ability of this compound to hydrogen bond to water through the unshared pair of electrons on the nitrogens, the compound is highly soluble in water. With functionalization of the purine ring, as in the case of adenine, guanine, and xanthine, the water solubility decreases. This is probably due to intramolecular interactions, which will be discussed in Chapter 18. Let it suffice to say that intramolecular interactions such as those shown in Figure 15-46 decrease the attractions that can occur with water. Finally, xanthine has both basic properties due to one of the nitrogens in the imidazole ring and acidic properties due to the imide NH in the pyrimidine ring.

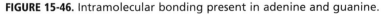

FIGURE 15-46. Intramolecular bonding present in adenine and guanine.

▪ **METABOLISM.** The metabolism of the substituted purine is quite systematic and is shown for adenine in Figure 15-47. The adenine is conjugated with 5-phosphoribosylpyrophosphate (PRPP) to give adenylic acid (adenosine-5′-phosphate). Adenylic acid in turn may be reduced to deoxyadenylic acid. A similar pattern of metabolism can lead to guanosine and xanthosine, which in turn can lead to guanylic acid and xanthylic acid.

A second type of metabolism common to purines is aromatic hydroxylation. An enzyme known as xanthine oxidase catalyzes this reaction. When xanthine is oxidized by xanthine oxidase, the resulting product is uric acid (Fig. 15-48).

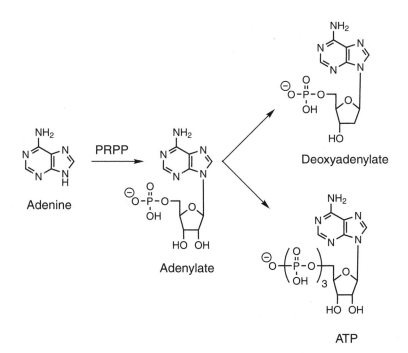

FIGURE 15-47. Metabolism of adenine.

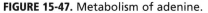

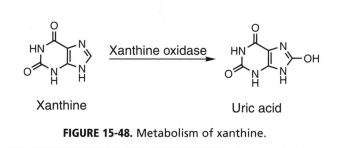

FIGURE 15-48. Metabolism of xanthine.

BICYCLIC HETEROCYCLES: SIX-MEMBERED RING PLUS SIX-MEMBERED RING

One Nitrogen

■ **NOMENCLATURE.** Two important bicyclic heterocycles containing a nitrogen in two fused six-membered rings are quinoline and isoquinoline (Fig. 15-49). These nuclei are common to synthetic and naturally occurring drugs. The rings are numbered as shown. The bridgehead positions are not numbered.

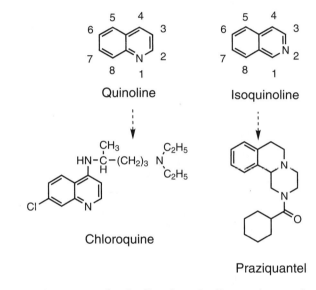

FIGURE 15-49. Structures of quinoline, isoquinoline, and examples of drugs containing these nuclei.

■ **PHYSICAL-CHEMICAL PROPERTIES.** Both quinoline and isoquinoline are weak bases similar to pyridine. These weak bases react with a strong acid such as sulfuric acid or hydrochloric acid to form water-soluble salts. Both compounds are aromatic and therefore have few additional properties that need concern us.

■ **METABOLISM.** The common metabolism seen in quinolines and isoquinolines is aromatic hydroxylation at one of the positions occupied by hydrogen.

One Oxygen

■ **NOMENCLATURE.** Another important bicyclic heterocycle found in nature and several synthetic drugs is the coumarin molecule (Fig. 15-50). Although the compound possesses a more complicated official name, the common name is usually used.

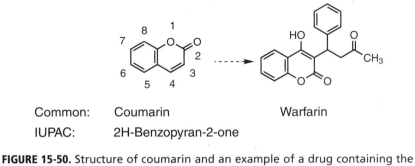

Common: Coumarin   Warfarin

IUPAC: 2H-Benzopyran-2-one

FIGURE 15-50. Structure of coumarin and an example of a drug containing the coumarin nucleus.

■ **PHYSICAL-CHEMICAL PROPERTIES.** The coumarin molecule contains an intramolecular ester known as a lactone. Lactones experience the same types of instabilities as esters. Lactones are prone to hydrolysis catalyzed by either acid or base to give a carboxylic acid and phenol (Fig. 15-51) (see Chapter 12 and Fig. 12-2)

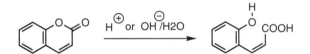

FIGURE 15-51. Acid- or base-catalyzed hydrolysis of coumarin.

■ **METABOLISM.** Esterase-catalyzed hydrolysis of coumarins would be expected to occur in the body, the product being the more soluble carboxylic acid shown in Figure 15-51.

Two or More Nitrogens

■ **NOMENCLATURE.** Two additional bicyclic heterocycles that serve as nuclei for several synthetic drugs and natural products are quinazoline and pteridine (Fig. 15-52).

■ **PHYSICAL-CHEMICAL PROPERTIES.** The properties of quinazoline and pteridine are similar to the monocyclic six-membered heterocycles. Both compounds are aromatic and possess basic nitrogens. Like pyridine or pyrimidine, the nitrogens are weak bases and therefore form salts in the presence of a strong acid.

■ **METABOLISM.** The metabolism expected for both quinazoline and pteridine is aromatic hydroxylation. This can occur at any of the positions occupied by a hydrogen.

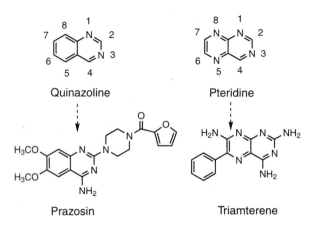

Quinazoline   Pteridine

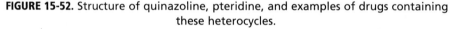

Prazosin   Triamterene

FIGURE 15-52. Structure of quinazoline, pteridine, and examples of drugs containing these heterocycles.

Two Nitrogens Plus Sulfur

■ **NOMENCLATURE.** While there are many additional bicyclic six-plus-six hetero-cyclics containing a variety of heteroatoms with various arrangements of the heteroatoms, one additional nucleus worth mentioning is the benzothiadiazine-1,1-dioxide shown in Figure 15-53. This nucleus is important as it serves as the base for the thiazide diuretics.

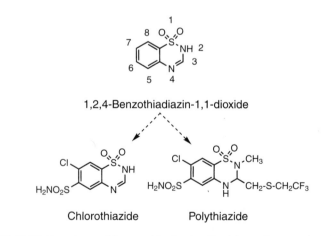

1,2,4-Benzothiadiazin-1,1-dioxide

Chlorothiazide   Polythiazide

FIGURE 15-53. Structure of benzothiadiazinedioxide and examples of drugs containing this heterocycle.

■ **PHYSICAL-CHEMICAL PROPERTIES.** A recognition of the functionality of this nucleus dictates the properties of the molecule. Present in the benzothiadiazine are a basic nitrogen and a cyclic sulfonamide (Fig. 15-54). The basic nitrogen is a

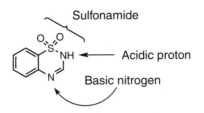

FIGURE 15-54. Functional groups and properties of a thiazide nucleus.

relatively weak base. Depending on whether the sulfonamide nitrogen is substituted or not determines whether this group is acidic or neutral. The unsubstituted sulfonamide nitrogen imparts acidic properties, while substitution at this nitrogen removes the acidic characteristics.

▪ **METABOLISM.** No unique metabolic properties are found with this nucleus.

BICYCLIC HETEROCYCLES: SIX-MEMBERED RING PLUS SEVEN-MEMBERED RING

Two Nitrogen Atoms

▪ **NOMENCLATURE.** An important six-plus-seven fused bicyclic heterocycle will be encountered in medicinal chemistry. This system is referred to generically as the benzodiazepine class of drugs (Fig. 15-55). The official nomenclature indicates that

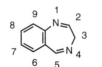 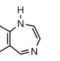 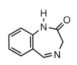

3H-1,4-Benzodiazepine   1H-1,4-Benzodiazepine   1,3-Dihydro-2H-1,4-Benzodiazepin-2-one

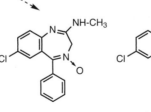 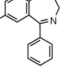

Chlordiazepoxide   Diazepam

FIGURE 15-55. Structure of 1,4-benzodizaepines and examples of drugs containing this heterocycle.

a benzene ring ("benzo") has been fused to a seven-membered ring ("pine"), which in turn contains two nitrogens ("diaz"). The 1,4- designates the location of the two nitrogen atoms. Since a seven-membered ring can accommodate only three double bonds, the 3H tells indirectly that with a hydrogen at the 3 position, the double bonds are at the site of ring fusion as well as at the 1,2 and 4,5 positions. An alternate arrangement of double bonds is shown for 1H-1,4-benzodiazepine. While 3H-1,4-benzodiazepine is the basic nucleus for the drug chlordiazepoxide, most of the benzodiazepines fall into the class of 1,3-dihydro-2H-1,4-benzodiazepin-2-ones. This heterocycle has an amide group present at the 1,2 position, with the carbonyl ("one") being present at the 2 position. The numbering system for the benzodiazepines is as shown.

■ PHYSICAL-CHEMICAL PROPERTIES. Few distinctive properties of the benzodiazepines need concern us. The nitrogen at the 4 position is a basic, but only weakly basic, nitrogen. Salt formation at this position to give a water-soluble salt is usually not practiced, probably because of the weakness of this base. The nitrogen at the 1 position is weakly basic in the 3H-1,4-benzodiazepine and neutral in the amide 1,4-benzodiazepin-2-one structure.

■ METABOLISM. Extensive data are available on the metabolism of the benzodiazepines. In many cases, the metabolism involves the additional substituents normally attached to the benzodiazepine nucleus. Metabolism of specific drugs will be discussed in the medicinal chemistry course. A common metabolic process that involves the 1,3-dihydro-2H-1,4-benzodiazepin-2-one nucleus is hydroxylation of the 3 position. This is seen with many of the anti-anxiety drugs.

TRICYCLIC HETEROCYCLES

■ NOMENCLATURE. A wide variety of tricyclic heterocycles, some of which are of medicinal significance, might be presented. Three representative nuclei are shown in Figure 15-56: phenothiazine, dibenzazepine, and acridine. The nomenclature and numbering of these heterocycles are as shown. Note that the numbering system for each of these compounds is unique.

■ PHYSICAL-CHEMICAL PROPERTIES. The phenothiazine nucleus contains a nitrogen that should be considered nearly neutral. Two aromatic rings attached to a nitrogen, each withdrawing electrons, reduce the basic property significantly. In most cases, this nitrogen will not form a salt with acid. The same reasoning holds for the nitrogen in 5H-dibenz[b,f]azepine. Acridine, although a weak base, can form salts with a strong acid.

An interesting physical property of the phenothiazine nucleus is that the molecule is not flat (Fig. 15-57). The shape of this molecule is thought to affect its biologic activity, and the amount of bend from planarity therefore may be important.

A characteristic of the acridine nucleus is the fact that the molecule possesses color. The nature of the color depends upon the substituents added to the three

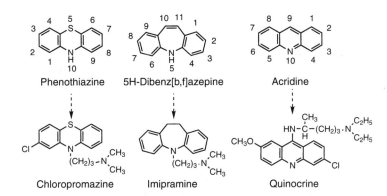

Phenothiazine   5H-Dibenz[b,f]azepine   Acridine

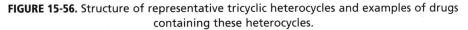

Chloropromazine   Imipramine   Quinocrine

FIGURE 15-56. Structure of representative tricyclic heterocycles and examples of drugs containing these heterocycles.

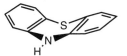

FIGURE 15-57. Conformational structure of phenothiazine.

rings. The fact that a molecule possesses color indicates a highly conjugated molecule with alternating single and double bonds. With three conjugated rings, a yellow coloration is seen.

■ **METABOLISM.** The characteristic metabolism found in all three of the tricyclic compounds is aromatic hydroxylation. Since the medicinally useful agents have substitution on these nuclei, the substitution will influence the site of hydroxylation.

An additional metabolism common to the phenothiazine nucleus is oxidation of the sulfur to the sulfoxide or sulfone. This reaction can be expected for any thioether and was discussed previously (see Fig. 14-2)

Oligonucleotides and Nucleic Acids

By far the most important chemicals in all living cells are the nucleic acids deoxyribonucleic acid (DNA) and ribonucleic acid (RNA). These polymeric molecules are the sources of all information needed for the construction of a living organism and the production of the proteins that run the organism, respectively. DNA found in the nucleus of eukaryotic cells is a double-stranded polymer that makes up the genes of an organism. DNA uncoils into a "sense" strand of nucleic acid and an "antisense" strand. The "antisense" strand is transcribed into messenger RNA (mRNA), which has the same sequence as the "sense" strand of DNA. The mRNA leaves the nucleus and in the ribosome serves as the template defining the sequence for protein synthesis. Thus, DNA and its messenger RNA prescribe the construction of all of the proteins of the body that carry out the day-to-day function of the living organism.

■ **NOMENCLATURE.** The two nucleic acids, DNA and RNA, are made up of four heterocyclic bases: guanine, adenine, and cytosine (common to both DNA and RNA) and uracil or thymine, present in RNA and DNA, respectively (Fig. 16-1). As discussed in Chapter 15, guanine and adenine are purines, while cytosine, uracil, and thymine are pyrimidines. Two pentoses are present in the nucleic acids, and these pentoses are ribose or deoxyribose in RNA or DNA, respectively. When the pentoses are attached to the N-9 position of the purines or the N-1 position of the pyrimidines, the resulting product is named a *nucleoside*. The suffix "-side" indicates the presence of a sugar. Attachment of the sugar to the bases occurs at the 1' position of the sugar. The linkage between the sugar and the heterocyclic base is through an acetal functional group. Finally, a phosphoric acid is added to the 5' position of the pentose to give the nucleotide. The phosphate attachment to the sugar is considered an ester group. Nucleic acids result from the polymerization of nucleotides through ester formation of the 5'-phosphate to the 3' alcohol of the pentose (Fig. 16-2). The continuous chain of pentose-3',5'-diester is present as the backbone to this polymer.

An oligonucleotide is a short-chain polymer of nucleotides with the same three components: base, sugar, and phosphate ester. The significance of oligonucleotides is that they represent a new approach to drug therapy, and such agents are referred to as "antisense drugs." Such drugs are designed to block protein synthesis in diseases associated with an abnormal protein and overexpression of a normal protein. The antisense drug is designed to interact with mRNA through Watson-Crick base pairing, leading ultimately to the blockage or termination of the action of mRNA.

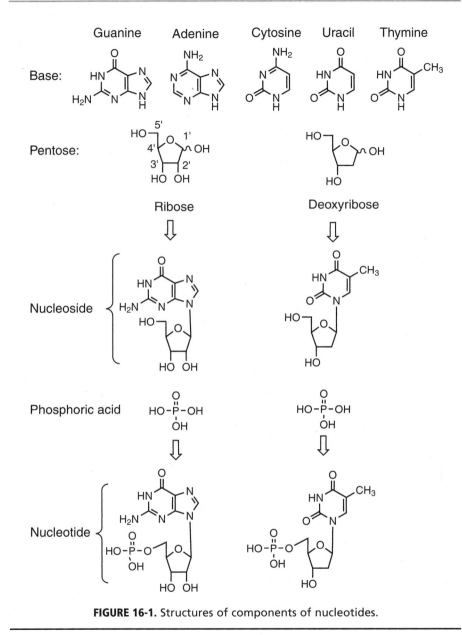

FIGURE 16-1. Structures of components of nucleotides.

The nomenclature used to identify the length of an oligonucleotide is to use an Arabic number corresponding to the number of nucleotides present, followed by "mer." Thus, the presence of 21 nucleotides would be to indicate the compound as a 21-mer oligonucleotide.

▪ **PHYSICAL-CHEMICAL PROPERTIES.** The most significant physical-chemical properties possessed by oligonucleotides and nucleic acids are their hydrophilic-

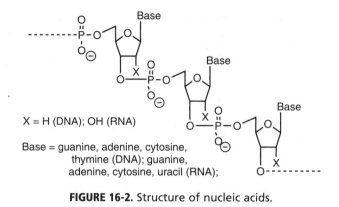

X = H (DNA); OH (RNA)

Base = guanine, adenine, cytosine,
thymine (DNA); guanine,
adenine, cytosine, uracil (RNA);

FIGURE 16-2. Structure of nucleic acids.

lipophilic properties and the ability of the various bases to recognize each other through hydrogen bonding. The backbone of the nucleotide diesters is hydrophilic in nature. At biologic pH, the phosphate diester is in an ionic state capable of ion-dipole bonding to water, and the pentose has hydrophilic character. The bases are usually considered hydrophobic in nature (Fig. 16-3).

The most unusual characteristic of nucleotides is the ability of the various bases to base pair through hydrogen bonding. The Watson-Crick model states that a guanine will base pair to a cytosine through three hydrogen bonds, while an adenine will base pair to thymine through two hydrogen bonds (Fig. 16-4). This base pairing in DNA thus results in the double helix, in which the ratio of guanine to cytosine is always 1 and the ratio of adenine to thymine is always 1. Because of the base pairing of the two strands of DNA, the hydrophobic bases are oriented to the inside of the double helix and the hydrophilic backbone is oriented to the outside of the helix.

Unlike DNA, RNA tends to exist as single strands with intermittent intramolecular base pairing, resulting in the formation of loops in the structure.

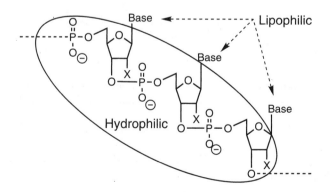

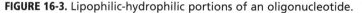

FIGURE 16-3. Lipophilic-hydrophilic portions of an oligonucleotide.

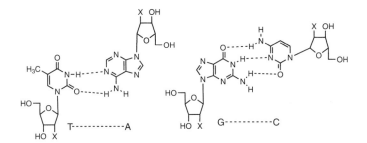

FIGURE 16-4. Base pairing of thymine (T) to adenine (A) and guanine (G) to cytosine(C).

The design of oligonucleotide drugs (antisense drugs) is based upon the fact that deoxyribonucleotide analogs can base pair to complementary areas in mRNA and as a result can bind to a specific region of the mRNA to disrupt protein synthesis. This does require that one identify stretches of mRNA that are not base paired and that the chosen mRNA be associated with the aberrant protein.

Oligonucleotides present an in vitro stability problem in that they are prone to both acid- and base-catalyzed hydrolysis. The site most likely to undergo hydrolysis is at the phospho diester bond. The hydrolytic process leads to formation of oligonucleotide fragments, with a phosphate ester remaining at either the 3′ or 5′ position of the pentose. An interesting complication to the base-catalyzed hydrolysis of ribose-containing oligonucleotides has been seen. The ribose oligonucleotides are more likely to undergo base-catalyzed hydrolysis than their deoxyribose counterpart due to the participation of the 2′-OH in the hydrolysis reaction (Fig. 16-5).

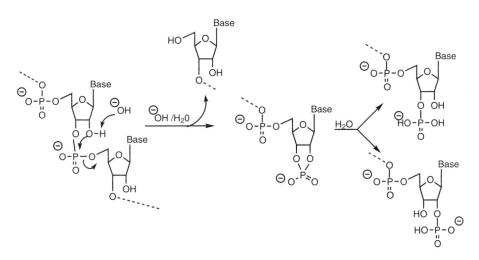

FIGURE 16-5. Base catalyzed hydrolysis of a ribose oligonucleotide.

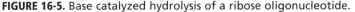

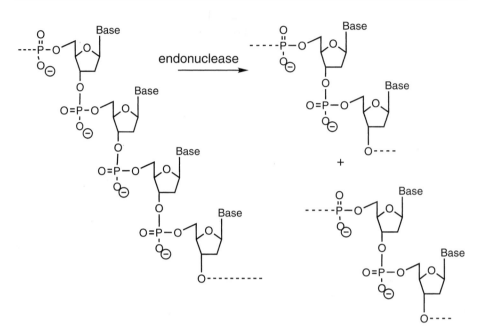

FIGURE 16-6. Metabolism of an oligonucleotide by endonuclease.

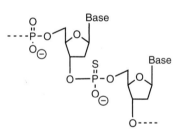

Phosphorothioate

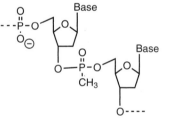

Methylphosphonate

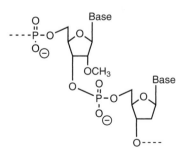

2'-O-Methylribonucleotide

FIGURE 16-7. Structural modification of oligonucleotides to protect against nuclease metabolism.

■ **METABOLISM.** Common metabolism of oligonucleotides and nucleic acids is via nuclease enzymes. Such enzymes are common to most tissues of the body, and they can attack terminal phosphodiester bonds (exonucleases) or internal phosphodiester bonds (endonucleases) to break the backbone of the oligonucleotide or nucleic acid (Fig. 16-6). The design of nuclease-resistant drugs has turned to modification of the backbone of the oligonucleotide through changes in the structure of the phosphodiester or changes in the pentose. Examples of the former are phosphorothioates and methylphosphonates, while an example of the latter would be 2′-O-methylribonucleotide (Fig. 16-7). Such derivatives show increased stability toward cellular nucleases.

Proteins

Another of the important macromolecules present in biologic systems are the polymers composed of amino acids and termed *proteins*. Derived from the Greek word *proteios* ("of the first order"), proteins have always occupied a significant niche in biochemistry instruction. From a pharmacologic standpoint, proteins have been recognized for their importance as enzymes catalyzing the reactions of the cell. They serve as key components of many, if not most, drug receptor sites. They have an important role in drug transport, and they have biologic activity as hormones. These naturally occurring materials may be relatively small molecules consisting of a few amino acids (Fig. 17-1) to extremely large-molecular-weight compounds made up of hundreds of amino acids. In the past, medicinal chemistry coverage of proteins has been limited because only a few protein drugs were available and the complexity of their synthesis, purification, chemistry, and administration made an in-depth discussion difficult and unproductive. With the recent discoveries in recombinant DNA technology, methods in hybridoma technology, automated protein synthesis, and newer methods of drug delivery, however, proteinaceous drugs are now not only possible but in fact have begun to appear on the market, with the expectation that scores of additional drugs will appear in the near future. As a result it is extremely important to be familiar with the basic chemical features of protein stability in vitro as well as potential protein metabolism.

■ **NOMENCLATURE.** Naturally occurring proteins are made up of 20 amino acids. These 20 amino acids are linked through amide bonds into a polymeric structure called a polypeptide or the protein. The arrangement of the amino acids within the protein is determined by the organism's DNA structure, as translated by messenger RNA (mRNA). The amino acids making up the protein may be neutral, acidic, or basic amino acids (Table 17-1).

The arrangement of amino acids in the protein gives the primary structure of the protein. The three-dimensional structure of a protein (that is, how it is arranged in space) will define the protein's secondary, tertiary, or quaternary structure, The spatial arrangements of a protein are discussed in detail in *Foye's Principles of Medicinal Chemistry*, Chapter 6. The presentation of a protein structure may appear in various forms, examples of which are shown in Figure 17-1. Commonly, the structure is shown using the abbreviations for the various amino acids, since the other representations are difficult to interpret and to draw.

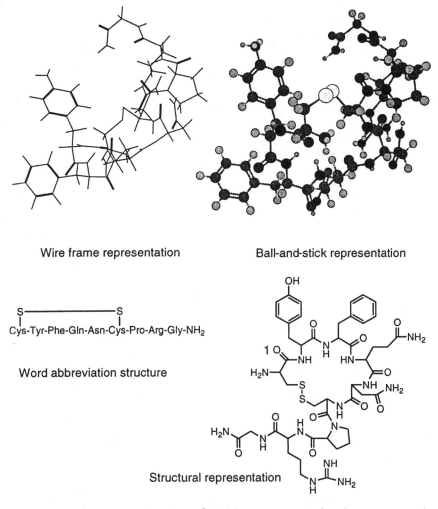

Wire frame representation   Ball-and-stick representation

Word abbreviation structure

Structural representation

FIGURE 17-1. Various representations of arginine vasopressin (AVP), a nonapeptide.

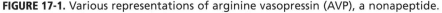

▪ **PHYSICAL-CHEMICAL PROPERTIES.** Although several unique physical-chemical properties are associated with proteins, some properties are predictable based upon the properties of the monomers that make up the polymeric macromolecules. The individual units that constitute the structure of proteins are the 20 amino acids, 19 of which are chiral molecules possessing the L-configuration. Amino acids are characteristically hydrophilic; this same property is found in proteins. Because of this hydrophilic nature, proteins tend to show poor penetration through lipophilic membranes, such as the intestinal lining, cell membranes, and blood-brain barrier.

Chemical instability of proteins follows a pattern related to the functionality of the individual amino acids present in the protein. The general types of chemical

Table 17-1. STRUCTURES OF NATURAL AMINO ACIDS

$$R \overset{COOH}{\underset{H_2N \quad H}{\diagup}}$$

Amino acid	Abbreviation	Structure R =
Neutral:		
Glycine	Gly, G	H
Alanine	Ala, A	CH_3
Isoleucine	Ile, I	$C_2H_5-\overset{CH_3}{\underset{H}{C}}-$
Leucine	Leu, L	$H_3C-\overset{CH_3}{\underset{H}{C}}-CH_2-$
Valine	Val, V	$H_3C-\overset{CH_3}{\underset{H}{C}}-$
Cysteine	Cys, C	$HS-CH_2-$
Methionine	Met, M	$H_3C-S-CH_2\cdot CH_2-$
Serine	Ser, S	$HO-CH_2-$
Threonine	Thr, T	$H_3C-\underset{OH}{CH}-$
Asparagine	Asn, N	$H_2N-\overset{O}{C}-CH_2-$
Glutamine	Gln, Q	$H_2N-\overset{O}{C}-(CH_2)_2^-$
Phenylalanine	Phe, F	⬡$-CH_2-$
Tryptophan	Trp, W	(indole ring)$-CH_2-$
Proline	Pro, P	(pyrrolidine ring with $-COOH$)
Acidic:		
Aspartic acid	Asp, D	$HO-\overset{O}{C}-CH_2-$
Glutamic acid	Glu, E	$HO-\overset{O}{C}-(CH_2)_2^-$
Tyrosine	Tyr, Y	$HO-$⬡$-CH_2-$
Basic:		
Arginine	Arg, R	$H_2N-\overset{NH}{\underset{}{C}}-\underset{H}{N}-(CH_2)_3-$
Lysine	Lys, K	$H_2N-(CH_2)_4-$
Histidine	His, H	(imidazole ring)$-CH_2-$

reactions seen in proteins consist of oxidation-reduction, deamidation, hydrolysis, and racemization reactions.

Oxidation Reactions. The amino acids most prone to oxidation reactions consist of methionine (Met), cysteine (Cys), histidine (His), tryptophan (Try), and Tyrosine (Tyr). The amino acid methionine contains a thioether functional group (Fig. 17-2). This unit is readily oxidized by mild oxidizing agents, such as hydrogen peroxide, as well as oxygen in the air, and represents a potential problem for storage of proteins.

The amino acid cysteine contains the thiol functional group, which is also readily oxidized to any of a number of oxidation states, depending on the strength of the oxidizing agent. Potentially the simplest oxidation may be the conversion of the thiol to a disulfide (cystine), a reaction that occurs in the presence of oxygen and metal ions (Fig. 17-3). The reverse of this reaction (that is, the reduction of a disulfide linkage of cystine) may also occur readily during protein isolation and purification. Since intramolecular and intermolecular disulfide bonds are common in proteins, a reduction of the disulfide bond will result in significant changes in the physical-chemical properties of the protein as well as the biologic activity of the protein. The disulfide bond forces the protein to adopt a specific shape, and thus breaking this bond allows the molecule to "unfold" and take on a new shape, which results in totally different properties. Disulfide bonds are quite common in biologically active proteins including molecules such as vasopressin (see Fig. 17-1), somatostatin, oxytocin, parathyroid hormone, and insulin.

The oxidation of histidine, tryptophan, and tyrosine has been reported to occur with a variety of oxidizing agents. In those cases in which oxidation occurs, it is

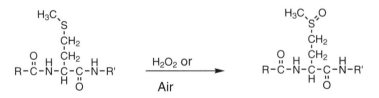

FIGURE 17-2. Oxidation of methionine.

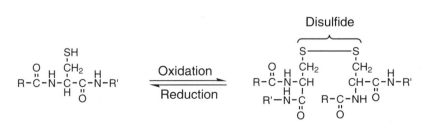

FIGURE 17-3. Oxidation of cysteine, reduction of cystine.

thought that the aromatic ring is cleaved, but structures of the breakdown products have not been characterized. With histidine and tryptophan, it is postulated that the products of oxidation are aspartic acid and N-formyl kynurenine, respectively (Fig. 17-4).

Deamidation Reactions. A common in vitro reaction of asparagine (Asn) and possibly of glutamine (Gln) is the hydrolysis of the side chain amide. This reaction has been investigated extensively for asparagine, with the nature of the products being influenced by the pH of the medium. If the pH is strongly acidic, a simple hydrolysis occurs, resulting in formation of the aspartyl peptide (Fig. 17-5). When the protein is stored at neutral or alkaline pH, not only is the aspartyl peptide produced but in addition the isoaspartyl peptide can be isolated. This reaction has been shown to proceed through a cyclic imide intermediate that opens readily to give the two possible products (see Fig. 17-5). These changes can be expected to

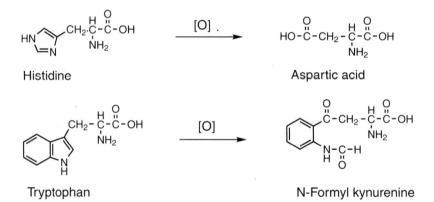

Histidine   Aspartic acid

Tryptophan   N-Formyl kynurenine

FIGURE 17-4. Oxidation of histidine and tryptophan.

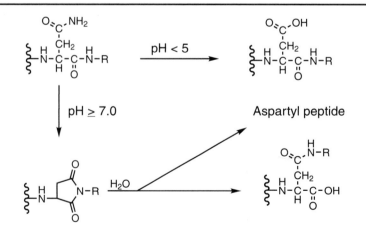

pH < 5

Aspartyl peptide

pH ≥ 7.0

H₂O

FIGURE 17-5. Deamidation of asparagine-containing protein at acidic or basic pH.

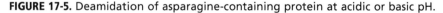

have a profound effect on the physical-chemical properties and the biologic activity of the modified protein.

A similar process can be invoked for hydrolysis of the glutamine side chain, but at present there is little supportive chemical evidence to suggest that this reaction is a serious problem in vitro.

Hydrolysis Reaction. Hydrolysis of peptide bonds in a protein generally does not occur. The typical amide bond is relatively stable with one exception. An aspartate (Asp) residue in the protein greatly increases the potential for hydrolysis of the peptide at the N-terminal and/or C-terminal position of this amino acid at acidic pH. The presence of a side chain carboxyl is important since this group assists the hydrolysis reaction, as shown in Figure 17-6. The hydrolysis obviously results in destruction of the protein.

Racemization Reaction. Nineteen of the 20 amino acids contain a chiral center that in theory could be racemized under basic conditions to the D-enantiomer, thus resulting in a protein with large differences in physical-chemical properties and biologic activities. Most amino acids appear to be relatively stable to racemization, although some evidence suggests that aspartate residues may racemize through a cyclic imide (Fig. 17-7). The formation of the cyclic imide increases the ease of proton removal at the asymmetric carbon, which upon reprotonation leads to formation of both isomers. Presumably resonance stabilization of the α-carbanion in the imide plays an important role in the racemization reaction.

Conformational Changes. A unique property found in proteins, but not commonly found in the low-molecular-weight compounds previously dealt with, is the high degree of intramolecular and intermolecular bonding that occurs in proteins.

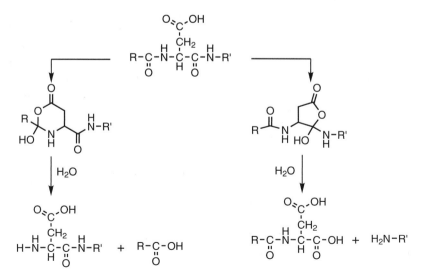

FIGURE 17-6. Hydrolysis of aspartate-containing protein.

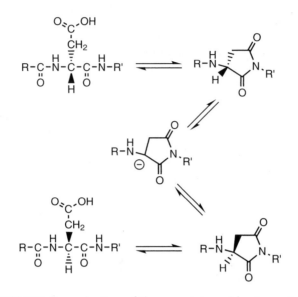

FIGURE 17-7. Racemization of the aspartate residue in proteins.

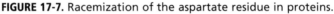

The amide functional groups found in protein can act as both a hydrogen donor and a hydrogen acceptor, leading to hydrogen bonding. If the hydrogen bonding occurs intramolecularly between the first and fourth peptide bond, the α-helix conformation results (Fig. 17-8), but if the hydrogen bonding occurs intermolecularly (or intramolecularly with a distant portion of the same protein), the β-sheet conformation is found (Fig. 17-9). The conformation of the protein resulting from the spatial arrangement and interactions due to nearby amino acids is referred to as the **secondary** structure of the protein. This secondary structure for the protein leads to a great deal of rigidity, but a rigidity that can be broken by temperature variations, changes in pH, or the presence of organic solvents. Molecules that are coiled or tightly packed due to hydrogen bonding have different physical-chemical and biologic properties than their nonbonded form. Another phenomenon seen with proteins is that they fold in such a way that the hydrophobic groups are buried in the interior of the polypeptide, while the hydrophilic groups are on the surface of the protein. The

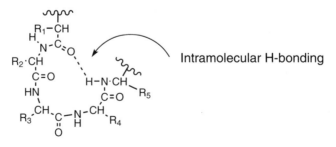

FIGURE 17-8. H-bonding resulting in an α-helix protein structure.

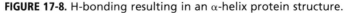

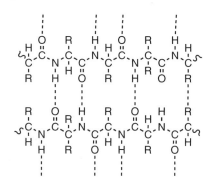

FIGURE 17-9. H-bonding resulting in a b-sheet protein structure.

protein becomes globular in structure. The globular long-distance conformation of a protein is referred to as the **tertiary** structure. Water binds readily to the protein, while van der Waals bonding occurs in the interior. This conformation of a protein confers specific physical-chemical and biologic activity to the protein. Once again, the globular conformation of the protein can be destroyed by temperature, pH, and solvent changes. The secondary and tertiary structures of the molecule are changed and the protein is said to be **denatured**. Unlike low-molecular-weight compounds, the polymeric proteins must be protected from drastic changes in temperature during storage, pH of the surrounding medium, and the presence of organic solvents.

▪ **METABOLISM.** A wide variety of metabolic reactions have been reported to occur in proteins, complicated to some extent by the fact that these reactions may be highly specific for a particular amino acid or for a certain dipeptide pattern. The types of metabolic reactions anticipated are oxidation-reduction reactions and hydrolysis reactions.

Oxidation Reductions. Similar to the oxidation reactions seen in vitro, it would be expected that methionine and cysteine would experience metabolic oxidation to give a sulfoxide and a disulfide, respectively (see Figs. 17-2 and 17-3). The resulting changes would be expected to produce proteins with physical-chemical properties and biologic activity quite different from those seen in the native protein. The oxidation of a cysteine to the disulfide or the reduction of a disulfide to the thiol of a cysteine changes the primary structure of a protein. For example, proteins containing disulfide bonds commonly have a cyclic structure (Fig. 17-10). If this bond is reduced, the cysteines, which were connected to each other (cystine), now may be separated by a great distance in the linear chain. The shape of the protein has undergone a drastic change and will lose whatever biologic activity it possessed. To return activity to a reduced protein requires oxidation of the thiol to the disulfide, and if several cysteines are present in the protein, an incorrect pairing may occur, leading to non-native protein with the incorrect three-dimensional structure.

Hydrolysis of Peptides. The breakdown of proteins under the influence of hydrolyzing enzymes can occur throughout the body. Intestinal fluids contain a

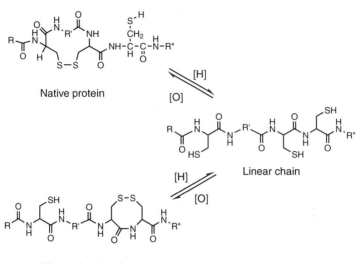

Native protein

Linear chain

Non-native protein

FIGURE 17-10. Reduction of the disulfide bond in a protein and oxidation of the thiol to the disulfide.

variety of peptidases, such as trypsin, chymotrypsin, elastase, and carboxypeptidase. Commonly found in the small intestine, these peptidases can completely degrade protein within a few minutes. But additionally, peptidases or their precursors may be found in the blood, in nerve synaptic regions, in the skin, and in fact in most fluids and tissues of the body. Therefore, the rapid metabolism of peptides can be expected, with the resulting termination of biologic activity.

A variety of aminopeptidases, carboxypeptidases, and deamidases attack and hydrolyze amide bonds. These enzymes may be highly selective for specific amino acids or combinations of amino acids. Table 17-2 lists the selectivity for several

Table 17-2. PROTEIN HYDROLYZING ENZYMES

Enzyme	Selectivity
Trypsin	Cleaves on carboxyl side of lysine and arginine
Thrombin	Cleaves arginine and glycine
Chymotrypsin	Cleaves on carboxyl side of aromatic amino acids (Tyr, Trp, Phe) and methionine
Pepsin	Cleaves tyrosine, tryptophan and phenylalanine
Carboxypeptidase A	Cleaves carboxy-terminal peptides (faster for aromatics and bulky aliphatic amino acids)
Carboxypeptidase B	Cleaves arginine and lysine
Elastase	Cleaves amide bonds of small and uncharged amino acids

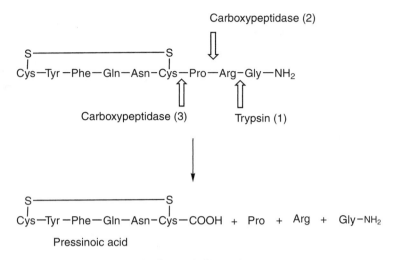

FIGURE 17-11. Intestinal metabolism of arginine vasopressin.

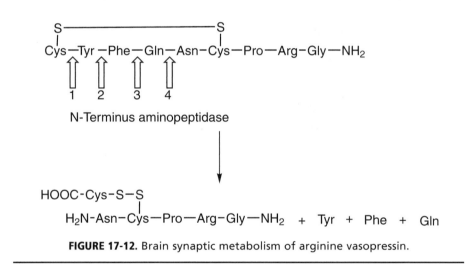

FIGURE 17-12. Brain synaptic metabolism of arginine vasopressin.

common enzymes. In general, aminopeptidase cleaves proteins starting at the N-terminal amino acid, carboxypeptidase cleaves amino acids from the C-terminal end of the peptide, and deamidases hydrolyze simple unsubstituted amides. As an example of the metabolism of a natural protein, Figure 17-11 outlines the metabolism of arginine vasopressin in intestinal juice, while Figure 17-12 indicates the metabolic fate of arginine vasopressin in brain synapses.

Predicting Water Solubility

EMPIRIC METHOD

We have now reviewed the major functional groups that might be expected in drug molecules. It will soon become obvious to you that the majority of the drugs discussed are not simple monofunctional molecules but instead are polyfunctional molecules. Most drugs will be found to contain two, three, four, or more of the organic functional groups within a single chemical entity. How, then, does one predict the physical and chemical properties of these more complex molecules?

As mentioned throughout the book, one must recognize the individual functional groups within the more complex structures. Once this is done, the chemical properties, namely in vitro stability and in vivo stability, are easily predicted. The chemical properties of a functional group are usually not affected by the presence of another functional group within the molecule. Therefore, each functional group can be treated independent of the other functional groups present.

If we consider the important physical property of water solubility, we find that polyfunctional molecules behave somewhat differently than monofunctional molecules. A simple summation of the water-solubilizing properties of each functional group usually does not lead to a successful prediction of water solubility for the more complex systems. With a single functional group, there is no possibility of intramolecular bonding (that is, bonding within the molecule) because no other functional group is present. On the other hand, with polyfunctional molecules, intramolecular bonding may become a significant interaction.

With the individual functional groups, intermolecular bonding is a factor in the solubilizing potential of the groups. For example, an alcohol functional group in a molecule such as hexanol binds to a second molecule of hexanol through dipole-dipole bonding. This bonding must be broken to dissolve the hexanol in water. When one states that an alcohol functional group solubilizes approximately six carbon atoms, one considers intermolecular bonding of this type. But what about the polyfunctional molecules? The intermolecular bonding between like functional groups can still occur, but now new types of bonding are possible. Bonding may occur between dissimilar functional groups of both an intermolecular and intramolecular type, and this bonding may be quite strong. For a molecule to dissolve in water, the intramolecular and intermolecular bonding must first be broken so that the water molecules can bond to the functional groups.

An excellent example of the importance of intramolecular bonding is seen with the amino acid tyrosine (Fig. 18-1). This molecule has three functional groups

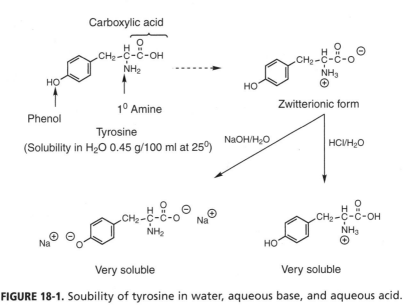

FIGURE 18-1. Soubility of tyrosine in water, aqueous base, and aqueous acid.

present: a phenol, an amine, and a carboxylic acid. By a simple summation of the water-solubilizing potential of each functional group, one would predict that the phenol would solubilize 6 or 7 carbon atoms, the amine 6 or 7 carbon atoms, and the carboxyl 5 or 6 carbon atoms, giving a total solubilizing potential of 17 to 20 carbon atoms. Tyrosine contains nine carbons, yet the molecule is soluble to the extent of 0.5%. The explanation for this lack of water solubility can be understood if one recognizes the possibility of intramolecular bonding. The amino acid can exist as a zwitterion (see Fig. 18-1). The charged molecule exhibits intramolecular ion-ion bonding, which destroys the ability of these two functional groups to bond to water. The phenol is not capable by itself of dissolving the molecule. If the intramolecular bonding is destroyed by adding either sodium hydroxide or hydrochloric acid to the amino acid, the resulting compound becomes quite water-soluble.

Most functional groups are capable of showing some intra- and intermolecular hydrogen bonding in a polyfunctional molecule, which decreases the potential for promoting water solubility. How much weight should be given to each such interaction for individual functional groups? This is a difficult question to answer, but as a general rule, if one is conservative in the amount of solubilizing potential that is given to each functional group, one will find that fairly accurate predictions can be made for polyfunctional molecules.

In Table 18-1, the various functional groups that have been discussed are listed with the solubilizing potential of each group when present in a monofunctional molecule and in a polyfunctional molecule. This latter value will be the more useful value, since most of the molecules that we discuss will be polyfunctional.

Several examples will help demonstrate this method of predicting water solubility. In the first example, Figure 18-2, one should recognize the presence of two

Table 18-1. WATER-SOLUBILIZING POTENTIAL OF ORGANIC FUNCTIONAL GROUPS WHEN PRESENT IN A MONO- OR POLYFUNCTIONAL MOLECULE. WATER SOLUBILITY IS DEFINED AS $>1\%$ SOLUBILITY

FUNCTIONAL GROUP	MONOFUNCTIONAL MOLECULE	POLYFUNCTIONAL MOLECULE
Alcohol	5 to 6 carbons	3 to 4 carbons
Phenol	6 to 7 carbons	3 to 4 carbons
Ether	4 to 5 carbons	2 carbons
Aldehyde	4 to 5 carbons	2 carbons
Ketone	5 to 6 carbons	2 carbons
Amine	6 to 7 carbons	3 carbons
Carboxylic Acid	5 to 6 carbons	3 carbons
Ester	6 carbons	3 carbons
Amide	6 carbons	2 to 3 carbons
Urea, Carbonate, Carbamate		2 carbons

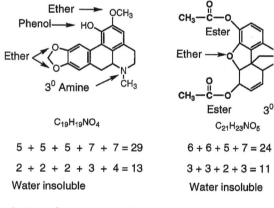

$C_{19}H_{19}NO_4$ $C_{21}H_{23}NO_5$

5 + 5 + 5 + 7 + 7 = 29   6 + 6 + 5 + 7 = 24

2 + 2 + 2 + 3 + 4 = 13   3 + 3 + 2 + 3 = 11

Water insoluble   Water insoluble

FIGURE 18-2. Prediction of water solubility of organic molecules using mono- and poly-functional estimates for the functional groups.

tertiary amines. If the more liberal solubilizing potential for an amine is used, it might be expected that each amine would have the capability of solubilizing up to 7 carbon atoms, leading to a total potential of dissolving 14 carbon atoms in the molecule. Since the molecule contains 13 carbon atoms, one would predict that the molecule would be soluble. Using the more conservative estimate and allowing three carbons worth of solubility to each amine, a prediction of insoluble would result. It turns out that the molecule *is* water-soluble. The use of the more liberal estimate to obtain the correct results is acceptable in this case because the molecule contains only amines that act alike, not creating any new inter- and intramolecular bonds. Probably also important for this molecule is the fact that both amines are tertiary amines, and tertiary amines cannot dipole-dipole bond to each other, and therefore intermolecular bonding is quite unlikely in this molecule.

With para-dimethylaminobenzaldehyde (see Fig. 18-2), a nine-carbon molecule, the liberal estimate would predict solubility, since the amine is capable of solubilizing up to seven carbon atoms and an aldehyde could solubilize up to five carbon atoms. On the other hand, the conservative estimate would predict insolubility, with the amine worth three and the aldehyde worth two carbon atoms. This molecule is listed as slightly soluble, a result that falls between the two estimates. This simply shows that these are only predictions and, with borderline compounds, may lead to inaccurate results.

The next examples shown in Figure 18-3 lead to a more accurate prediction. In the first compound in Figure 18-3, one should recognize the presence of three ethers, a phenol, and a tertiary amine. Using the monofunctional solubilizing potential, one would expect enough solubility from these groups to dissolve this 19-carbon compound, since each ether would be assigned 5 carbons, the phenol 7 carbons, and the amine 7 carbons worth of solubilizing potential. If one uses the more conservative estimate, which takes into consideration the intra- and intermolecular bonding, however, each ether contributes two carbons worth of solubility, while the phenol and amine contribute three and four carbons worth of solubilizing potential, respectively. The prediction now is that the molecule is insoluble in water, and this turns out to be the case.

The second structure in Figure 18-3 has two esters, an ether, and a tertiary amine. Once the functional groups are identified, one needs only to assign the solubilizing potential to each group. Again, the monofunctional potentials are inap-

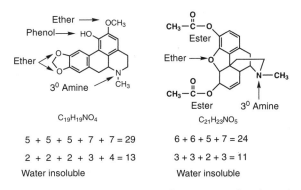

$C_{19}H_{19}NO_4$

5 + 5 + 5 + 7 + 7 = 29

2 + 2 + 2 + 3 + 4 = 13

Water insoluble

$C_{21}H_{23}NO_5$

6 + 6 + 5 + 7 = 24

3 + 3 + 2 + 3 = 11

Water insoluble

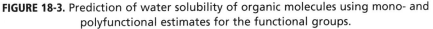

FIGURE 18-3. Prediction of water solubility of organic molecules using mono- and polyfunctional estimates for the functional groups.

propriate since this is a polyfunctional molecule, and if used would have resulted in a prediction of water solubility. Using the polyfunctional solubilizing potential gives the more accurate prediction of the molecule being water-insoluble. The polyfunctional potential is more appropriate since this molecule would be expected to have both intramolecular and intermolecular bonding.

Additional examples of the empiric approach to predicting water solubility can be found throughout the Functional Group Analysis Workbook.

ANALYTIC METHOD

Throughout this presentation, emphasis has been placed on the water-solubilizing properties of the common organic functional groups. This is restated in Table 18-1 with carbon-solubilizing potentials for each functional group; the use of these values was demonstrated by the examples shown in Figures 18-2 and 18-3. While this approach is empiric, others have attempted to derive an analytic method for calculation of water solubility. One such mathematical approach is based upon the partitioning of a drug between octanol (a standard for lipophilic media) and water. The base-ten logarithm of the partition coefficients is defined as log P. While the measured log P values are a measure of the solubility characteristics of the whole molecule, one can use fragments of the whole molecule and assign a specific hydrophilic-lipophilic value (defined as π value) to each of these fragments. Thus, a calculated log P can be obtained by the sum of the hydrophilic-lipophilic fragments:

$$\log P = \frac{\text{Conc. of Drug in Octanol}}{\text{Conc. of Drug in Water}} \qquad \text{(Eq. 1)}$$

$$\log P_{calc} = \Sigma \pi_{(fragments)} \qquad \text{(Eq. 2)}$$

To use this procedure, the student must fragment the molecule into basic units and assign an appropriate π value corresponding to the atoms or groups of atoms present. Table 18-2 lists the common fragments found in organic molecules and their π values. Positive values for π mean that the fragment, relative to hydrogen, is lipophilic or favors solubility in octanol. A negative value indicates a hydrophilic group and thus an affinity for water. While the environment of the substituent can influence the π value, such changes are small, and for our purposes this factor can be neglected.

Through the examination of a large number of experimentally obtained log P and solubility values, an arbitrary standard has been adopted whereby those chemicals with a positive log P value over +0.5 are considered water-insoluble (i.e., solubility is <3.3% in water—a definition for solubility used by the USP). Log P values less than +0.5 are considered water-soluble.

This method of calculating water solubility has proved quite effective with a large number of organic molecules containing C, Cl, N, and O, but several additional factors may have to be considered for specific drugs. A complicating factor is the influence of intramolecular hydrogen bonding (IMHB) on π values. As dis-

Table 18-2. HYDROPHILIC-LIPOPHILIC VALUES (π VALUES) FOR ORGANIC FRAGMENTS

Fragments	π Values
C (aliphatic)	+0.5
C (alkene)	+0.33
Phenyl	+2.0
Cl (halogen)	+0.5
S	+0.0
N (amine)	-1.0
O (hydroxyl, phenol, ether)	-1.0
O_2NO	+0.2
O_2N (aliphatic)	-0.85
O_2N (aromatic)	-0.28
O=C-O	-0.7
O=C-N (other than amine)	-0.7
IMHB	+0.65

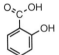

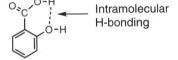 Intramolecular H-bonding

Solubility 0.2%

Calc. log P without IMHB		Calc. log P with IMHB	
Phenyl	+2.0	Phenyl	+2.0
O-H	-1.0	O-H	-1.0
O=C-O	-0.7	O=C-O	-0.7
		IMHB	+0.65
Total	+0.3	Total	+0.95
Prediction	Soluble	Prediction	Insoluble

FIGURE 18-4. Calculation of water solubility of salicylic acid without and with the intramolecular hydrogen bonding (IMHB) factor.

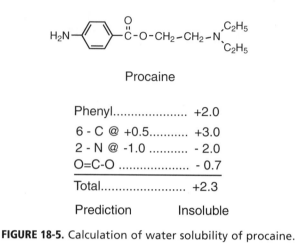

Procaine

Phenyl.....................	+2.0
6 - C @ +0.5...........	+3.0
2 - N @ -1.0	- 2.0
O=C-O	- 0.7
Total.......................	+2.3

Prediction   Insoluble

FIGURE 18-5. Calculation of water solubility of procaine.

cussed in the previous empiric approach to predicting water solubility, IMHB would be expected to decrease water solubility, and therefore where IMHB exists, a π value of +0.65 is added to the calculations. An example of using this factor is shown for salicylic acid (Fig. 18-4).

The log P values of a drug with acid or base character are influenced by the pH of the medium in which the drug is placed. This is not surprising, since acid or base groups will become ionic under appropriate conditions. Although the π values given in Table 18-2 were obtained under conditions in which the amine, phenol, or carboxylic acid are un-ionized, which would allow an accurate prediction of log P, observed log P's at various pH values may not be accurate for water prediction. The experimental log P's found for procaine are −0.32 (pH 7) and 0.14 (pH 8), both of which would lead to the prediction that procaine is water-soluble. In fact, procaine is soluble to the extent of 0.5% at pH 7. The calculated log P = +2.3 (Fig. 18-5) correctly predicts that procaine is water-insoluble.

Stereoisomerism—Asymmetric Molecules

A carbon atom with four different substituents does not possess a plane or point of symmetry and therefore is an asymmetric molecule. A carbon atom with two or more of the same substituents has either a plane or point of symmetry resulting in a symmetric molecule (Fig. A-1). For 2-methyl-2-butanol, carbon atoms 2, 3, and 4 and the OH lie in a plane with the methyls and hydrogens symmetrically located before and behind the plane. This compound has a plane of symmetry and is therefore a symmetric molecule. On the other hand, 2-butanol does not have a plane of symmetry, is asymmetric, and consists of two molecules or a pair of enantiomers. The second enantiomer can be easily generated by reflecting the molecule in a mirror, as shown in Figure A-2. If the mirror image is rotated 180°, one can see that the enantiomers are not superimposable. 2-Butanol is said to be a chiral molecule with two enantiomeric forms. What is the significance of chirality? The two enantiomers have the same empirical formula, and most physical-chemical properties are the same. The exception is that a chiral method of identification sees the two molecules as distinctly different. A common method of identifying enantiomers is by using plane polarized light. One of the isomers, when placed in a polarimeter, rotates the plane of polarization to the right (clockwise), is said to be dextrorotatory, and is labeled the d isomer or (+) isomer. The

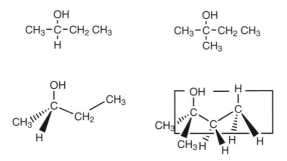

FIGURE A-1. Structure of the asymmetric 2-butanol and the summetric 2-methyl-2-butanol.

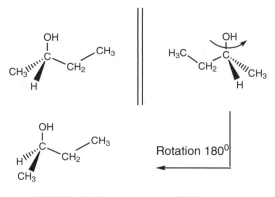

FIGURE A-2. Enantiomers of 2-butanol.

other isomer causes a counterclockwise rotation of the plane of polarization and is thus the levorotatory isomer, abbreviated as the l isomer or (-) isomer. The degree of rotation is the same for both enantiomers but in opposite directions. The fact that enantiomers can bend plane polarized light has caused such compounds to be referred to as optically active isomers. If a compound exists as an equal mixture of both isomers, the material is said to be racemic, with a net rotation of polarization of zero. Other chiral substances, important to medicinal chemistry, that can often distinguish between enantiomers with profound differences are biologic enzymes. Since enzymes are proteinaceous, they are made up of amino acids, which are chiral compounds. In the human body, enzymes are constructed of α-amino acids. Many chiral enzymes react selectively with one of the enantiomers of a chiral drug, producing a biologic response. The second enantiomer may have little or no biologic activity. One must recognize the presence of a chiral center in a drug molecule and appreciate the importance of this property as it affects biologic activity.

Finally, another aspect of a chiral center should be reviewed. The direction of rotation of plane polarized light is a relative property and does not indicate the absolute configuration around the chiral center. The Cahn-Ingold-Prelog "R" and "S" nomenclature is used to indicate absolute configuration. A set of arbitrary sequence rules assigns to the atoms around the chiral center priorities of 1 through 4, with number 1 being the highest priority. The molecule is then rotated so that the number 4 group is placed behind the remaining three groups and farthest from the eye. One then notes the direction in which the eye travels in going from 1 to 2 to 3. If the direction is clockwise, the molecule is assigned the absolute configuration of R, while if the direction is counterclockwise the center is assigned the S absolute configuration (Fig. A-3). While many sequence rules are used for the many different functional groups encountered in organic chemistry, the one that suffices for most situations is that the atom with a higher atomic number precedes

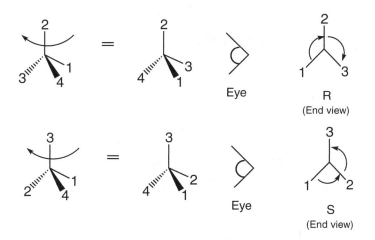

FIGURE A-3. Cahn-Ingold-Prelog method of assigning absolute configuration.

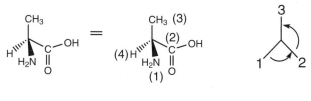

N > C-O > C-H > H

FIGURE A-4. (S)-2-aminopropionic acid [(S)-alanine].

a lower atomic number atom. Thus, for the amino acid alanine shown in Figure A-4, the N (atomic No. 7) has higher priority than C (atomic No. 6), which has higher priority than H (atomic No. 1). To differentiate between the CH$_3$ and the COOH group, one must go to the atoms attached to the carbons, and the O (atomic No. 8) has priority over H.

Acidity and Basicity

Throughout the book, considerable emphasis has been placed on the physical-chemical properties of the various functional groups. One of the major physical-chemical properties emphasized has been that of acidity/basicity. If a functional group is acidic, conversion of that group to a salt that can dissociate in water dramatically improves water solubility through ion-dipole bonding. In a similar fashion, if a functional group is basic, it can be converted to a salt by treatment with an acid. If the salt dissociates in water, water solubility will be increased through ion-dipole bonding. Since water solubility is quite important for drug delivery, it is felt that a short review of the concept of acidity and basicity is called for. In addition, a compilation of the important acids and bases, drawn from this book, will be presented in this appendix.

DEFINITIONS OF ACIDS AND BASES

Although there are several definitions for acids and bases, the most useful for our purposes is the Brønsted-Lowry definition. According to this definition, an acid is defined as any substance that can donate a proton; a base is a substance that can accept a proton. Shown here is the reaction of HX with water. HX is donating a proton to water, and HX is therefore an acid. By virtue of the fact that water is accepting the proton, water is a base. The anion, X^-, formed from the acid, HX, is also capable of accepting a proton and is thus defined as the conjugate base of HX. In a similar manner, the hydronium ion, H_3O^+, is a conjugate acid of the base water. In this reaction, there are two conjugate acid-base pairs: the conjugate acid-base pair made up of HX and X^- and the conjugate acid-base pair made up of H_2O and H_3O^+. The Brønsted-Lowry definition of acids and bases necessitates the concept of conjugate acid-base pairs. Indeed, an acid (or base) cannot demonstrate its acidic (or basic) properties unless a base (or acid) is present. In the example shown, HX cannot

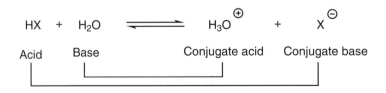

donate its proton unless there is another substance (a base) to accept that proton. Several additional examples of acids and bases are shown in Figure B-1.

Several interesting phenomena should be noted in these examples. Water is acting as a base in the first three examples and as an acid in the latter three examples. Since water can act as either an acid or a base, it is said to be amphoteric. Also seen in Figure B-1 are examples of compounds that demonstrate another useful definition of a base. Lewis defined a base as an electron-pair donor. This definition is useful in identifying organic bases such as amines. Alkyl and aryl amines are basic by virtue of their ability to donate a pair of electrons.

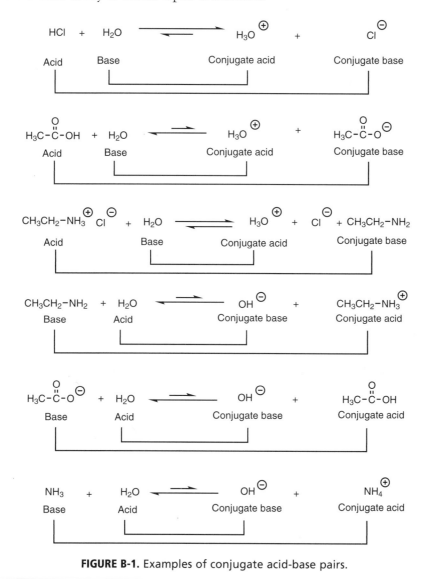

FIGURE B-1. Examples of conjugate acid-base pairs.

RELATIVE STRENGTHS OF ACIDS AND BASES

The strength of an acid depends on its ability to donate a proton. The strong acids have a strong tendency to give up a proton, while the weak acids have little tendency to give up a proton. Virtually all organic compounds could be considered acids. A compound like methane (CH_4) can give up a proton when treated with a sufficiently strong base. However, when dealing with water as the pharmaceutical solvent and with the intention of creating water-soluble salts, the list of acids is greatly reduced. Thus, the alcohol functional group, which an organic chemist may consider an acid, from our standpoint is considered a neutral functional group. The same limitations must be placed on the base. Many compounds that a chemist would consider basic will not give stable salts when placed in water. Therefore, the drug list of basic functional groups is quite limited.

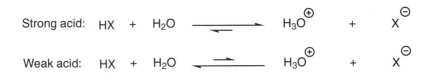

The discussion of the relative strength of an acid really becomes a discussion of the nature of the dissociation equilibrium for the acid in water. A strong acid is one that has a strong tendency to dissociate. The strong acids commonly used in pharmacy are nearly completely dissociated in water (e.g., H_2SO_4, HCl, HNO_3). If a compound is a strong acid, then its conjugate base is weak. The weak acids are

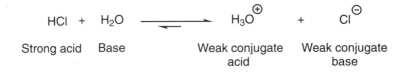

those compounds that have a poor tendency to dissociate in water (e.g., carboxylic acids, phenols, sulfonamides, imides). Such compounds are characterized as having relatively strong conjugate bases. In all cases, the equilibrium will tend to favor the direction that gives the weaker acid and the weaker base.

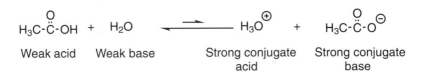

In a similar fashion, the relative strength of a base depends upon the ability of the chemical to give up a hydroxyl or the tendency to accept a proton. Table B-1 is a listing of common acids and bases in order of acidity. The table actually becomes compressed when water is specified as our solvent. All of the acids above the

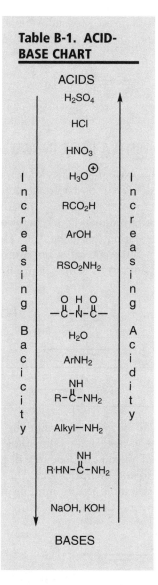

Table B-1. ACID-BASE CHART

hydronium ion show a reduction in apparent acidity because of the leveling effect in water. Since the strong acids (e.g., H_2SO_4, HCl, HNO_3) are nearly completely dissociated in water to form hydronium ions, their acidities become equal in water and the hydronium ion becomes the strongest ion. The leveling effect also affects strong bases. In water, the strongest base that can exist is the hydroxide ion; therefore, sodium hydroxide and potassium hydroxide, which completely dissociate, become equivalent in basicity.

A brief reminder about the acid-base properties of water, which can dissociate to form hydronium ion and hydroxide ion, is shown. The hydronium ions and hydroxide ions formed by this dissociation are present in equal concentrations (i.e., there is no excess of either hydronium ions or hydroxide ions). Hence, water is neutral.

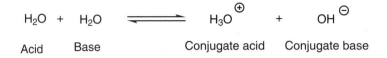

$$H_2O \ + \ H_2O \ \rightleftharpoons \ H_3O^{\oplus} \ + \ OH^{\ominus}$$

Acid   Base   Conjugate acid   Conjugate base

REACTION OF AN ACID WITH A BASE IN WATER

The reaction of an acid with a base in water is known as a neutralization reaction. When a strong acid reacts with a strong base, one actually finds that the reaction consists of hydronium ions formed by the acid reacting with the hydroxide ions formed by the base. The neutralization reaction between a strong acid and a strong base results in an aqueous solution that is neutral. The anion of an acid and the cation of a base do not react with each other but are simply present as a salt. The situation is not the same when a weak acid is neutralized by a strong base. In the

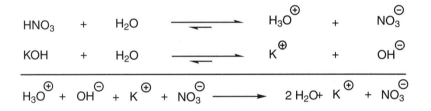

acid-base reaction between acetic acid and sodium hydroxide, sodium acetate, the weak conjugate base of acetic acid, and water, the weak conjugate acid of the hydroxide ion, are formed. The sodium acetate will partially dissociate in water, however, to afford acetic acid and hydroxide ion. This will result in a slight excess of hydroxide ion in solution when the "neutralization" reaction is complete, and the pH of the solution will be greater than 7, or alkaline.

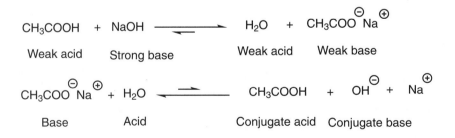

An analogous situation occurs in neutralization reactions between weak bases and strong acids, except that the final solution is acidic. In this example, the dissociation of the salt formed during the neutralization reaction produces hydronium ion. The resulting solution from this neutralization reaction will have a pH less than

7 (acidic), in that the strength of the hydronium ion is more acidic than the amine is basic. The amount of hydronium ion formed depends on the extent of dissociation of the amine salt.

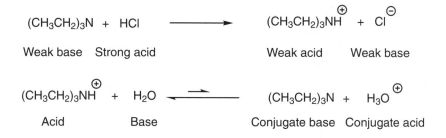

This concept is quite important if one considers what happens to the pH of water if a sodium or potassium salt of an organic acid is dissolved in water. The organic anion is the conjugate base of a weak acid, and when placed in water the pH of the solution becomes alkaline. Another way of considering this is that, in water, one has the salt of a weak acid and a strong base. Since the strong base is farther up the pH scale than the weak acid is down the scale, the net sum of this is that the pH remains greater than 7 (Fig. B-2). When a sulfate, chloride, or nitrate salt of an organic base is dissolved in water, one has a salt of a weak base and a strong acid. The strong acid is farther down the pH scale than the base is up the scale, and the pH of the solution therefore is below 7. Using this concept, one can successfully predict the pH of many salts after dissolving the salt in water (Table B-2). The clue to predicting the correct answer is in being able to recognize whether one is dealing with salts of strong acids and weak bases or weak acids and strong bases. A rule of thumb that is most helpful is that the strong acids are hydrochloric, sulfuric, nitric, perchloric, and phosphoric acid. All other acids are weak. The strong bases are sodium hydroxide and potassium hydroxide. All other bases are weak.

Salt of a strong base and a weak acid.

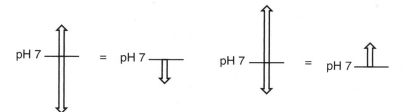

Salt of a strong acid and a weak base.

FIGURE B-2. Diagramatic representation for predicting pH of an aqueous media after addition of a water soluble salt to water.

Table B-2. DISSOCIATION IN WATER

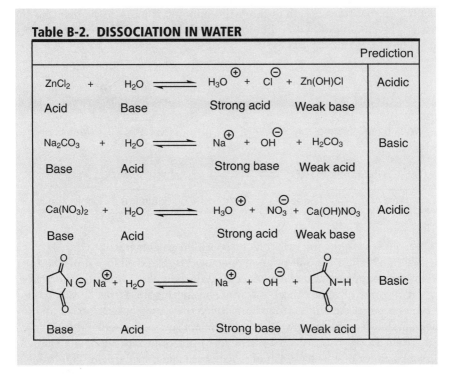

ACIDIC AND BASIC ORGANIC FUNCTION GROUPS

This section presents, in a single location, a synopsis of most of the organic acids and bases that are important in drugs as potential salt-forming sites. As stated earlier, nearly all organic compounds could be considered potentially acidic, but put in the context of water as the solvent, only a few functional groups are acidic enough to be of practical value.

Table B-3 lists the organic acids that have been reviewed in this book. Although sulfonic acids are the most acidic of the "organic" functional groups, few drugs contain them. The carboxylic acids are the most acidic organic functional groups found in drug molecules. The nature of the "R" group strongly influences the strength of this acidity (for a review of this influence, see Chap. 11).

When "R" is an electron-withdrawing group, relative to hydrogen, the acidity increases, and when "R" is an electron-releasing group, relative to hydrogen, the acidity decreases. The effects of "R" on acidity, inductively or by resonance, stabilize or destabilize the carboxylate anion, respectively. The sulfonamide is an acidic functional group provided that the sulfonamide is unsubstituted or monosubstituted. A disubstituted sulfonamide does not have a proton on the nitrogen and cannot be acidic. Phenols are relatively weak acids that can be strongly influenced by the nature of the aromatic substituent (see Chap. 7). Electron-withdrawing groups in

Table B-3. ORDER OF ACIDITY OF ORGANIC ACIDS

Acids	Acidity (pKa)
$R-SO_3H$	1
$R-COOH$	4 - 5
$Ar-SO_3NHR$	6 - 9
$Ar-OH$	8 - 11
(imide structure)	8 - 10

the para or meta position increase acidity by resonance or a combination of resonance and inductive action. Electron-releasing groups likewise reduce acidity because such groups destabilize the phenolate anion. Finally, common to a number of heterocycles is the imide functional group, which must have a proton on the nitrogen to be acidic.

All of the organic acids (with the exception of sulfonic acid) are weak acids, which is to say that, in water, the equilibrium will favor the undissociated molecule. This also explains why salts of organic acids and strong bases, when dissolved in water, produce an appreciable quantity of hydroxide ion, and the aqueous solution is alkaline. The degree of alkalinity will depend on the strength of the acid. Alkaline metal salts of phenols will result in a very basic aqueous solution, while alkaline metal salts of carboxylic acids are less basic.

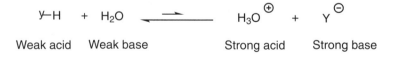

Y−H	+	H₂O		H₃O$^{\oplus}$	+	Y$^{\ominus}$
Weak acid		Weak base		Strong acid		Strong base

Table B-4 lists the organic bases that have been reviewed in this book. Guanidines are the most basic organic functional group, followed by the alkylamines. Within the class of alkylamines the usual order of basicity is secondary amines are more basic than tertiary amines, which are more basic than primary amines. Aromatic amines are significantly (10^{-10}) less basic than alkylamines (10^{-4}), owing to the fact that electron-releasing groups (alkyls) increase basicity, while electron-withdrawing groups (aryls) reduce basicity (see Chap. 10). Aromatic

Table B-4. ORDER OF BASICITY OF ORGANIC BASES

Bases	Basicity (pKa) (Conjugate acid)
$R \cdot HN - \overset{\overset{\textstyle NH}{\|}}{C} - NH_2$	~13
$R - NH_2$; $R_2 - NH$; $R_3 - N$	10 - 11
$R - \overset{\overset{\textstyle NH}{\|}}{C} - NH_2$	9 - 10
$Ar - NH_2$	1 - 5
	1 - 4

(Includes pyridine, imidazole, etc.)

heterocycles containing a nitrogen with a pair of nonbonding electrons are also basic; however, these compounds are weak bases.

$$B : \quad + \quad H_2O \quad \rightleftharpoons \quad BH^{\oplus} \quad + \quad OH^{\ominus}$$

Weak base   Weak acid   Strong acid   Strong base

All the organic bases are weak bases, which is to say that in water the equilibrium will favor the free base. Thus, when salts of the organic bases made with strong acids are dissolved in water, an appreciable quantity of hydronium ion will exist and the pH of the aqueous solution will be acidic, the degree of acidity depending on the strength of the base.

Drug Metabolism

INTRODUCTION

The biologic transformation of a drug molecule by enzymes present in the body is commonly referred to as drug metabolism. The process of drug metabolism is usually considered to be a process that leads to detoxification and increased water solubility. In actual fact, metabolism as a chemical transforming process can lead to an increase in toxicity, an activation or deactivation of the biologic action, and in some cases a decrease in water solubility. In addition, drugs represent only one small group of substrates that may undergo metabolism. Any substance foreign to the body can potentially be metabolized after entering the body. A more general term for exogenous substances is the term *xenobiotics*. Xenobiotics represent any foreign chemical and include intentional and unintentional food additives (i.e., herbicides and pesticides), volatile chemicals (i.e., substances in cigarette smoke), chemicals in the drinking water, environmental pollutants in the home and the workplace, as well as drugs. Finally, xenobiotic metabolism, while primarily occurring in the liver, may also occur at extrahepatic sites, including intestine (both within the lumen and the intestinal mucosa), kidney, lungs, nervous tissue, and plasma.

METABOLIC ENZYMES

Xenobiotic metabolism is generally divided into two types of reactions, referred to as phase 1 reactions and phase 2 reactions. Phase 1 reactions include oxidation, reduction, and hydrolysis reactions. These reactions generally involve introduction of a new functional group into the molecule. Phase 2 reactions, which normally follow phase 1, involve conjugation reactions such as acetylation, sulfation, glucuronidation, and conjugation with amino acids. Generally, conjugation reactions lead to inactivation of drug molecules. In many instances xenobiotic metabolism involves a combination of both phase 1 and phase 2 reactions. In any case, xenobiotic metabolism can be predicted and relies on the nature of the functional group or groups present in the organic molecule.

Oxygenase Enzymes

CYTOCHROME P450

A major oxidative enzyme system, and the most studied human enzyme system, is the cytochrome P450 monooxygenase family of enzymes (commonly abbreviated as CYP450). Found in the smooth endoplasmic reticulum of the liver, as well as in some extrahepatic tissue, CYP450 is a very complex enzyme made up of iron-protoporphyrin, NADPH, flavin protein, phospholipids, phosphatidylcholine, and molecular oxygen. CYP450 monooxygenase is not a single enzyme, but instead a family of closely related isoforms. A large number of different isoforms of CYP450 have been identified, each showing a different degree of selectivity and range of activity towards various xenobiotics. It appears that at least eight isoforms of CYP450 play important roles in drug metabolism. Genetic variation appears to play a role in defining the content of each isoform present in human beings and may account for the variations and extent of drug metabolism seen in individual patients. Scientists are just beginning to understand and characterize the structural requirements for selectivity associated with the isoforms of CYP450. The emerging area of pharmacogenomics (that is, the selection of the right drug for the right patient) can be expected to rely heavily on defining the genetic makeup of CYP450 isoforms of individuals. For a more detailed look at this family of enzymes, their mechanisms of metabolism, and the potential for drug-drug interaction, the reader is referred to *Foye's Principles of Medicinal Chemistry*, 5th edition, Chapter 8.

CYP450 CATALYZED REACTIONS

The common metabolic oxidation reactions involving CYP450 are shown in Table C-1. Oxidation of hydrocarbons is usually dependent upon the nature of the hydrocarbon. While aromatic hydroxylation is quite common, the oxidation of an alkane or alkene is not very common. Oxidation of the alkane carbon adjacent to an aromatic ring is more likely to occur than other sites of alkane oxidation. Alkene metabolism of natural substrates is more likely than is oxidation of alkene xenobiotics.

Dealkylation of short straight chain ethers and amines is a common reaction catalyzed by CYP450. In the case of ethers, it is common for methyl, ethyl, or propyl aryl ethers to be dealkylated, giving rise to phenols and formaldehyde, acetylaldehyde, or propanaldehyde, respectively. Primary amines undergo deamination, while secondary and tertiary short chain amines undergo dealkylation, giving ammonia, a primary amine, or a secondary amine, respectively. Deamination and dealkylation are both identical processes.

Finally, thioethers are oxidized by CYP450 enzymes, leading to a sulfoxide, a single oxidation, or a sulfone, a second oxidation. While thioethers are prone to this type of oxidation, CYP450 is not the usual catalyst for this reaction (see below).

Since the CYP450 family of enzymes are common metabolizing enzymes for a wide variety of xenobiotics, it should not be surprising to find drug-drug, drug-food, and drug-environmental chemical interactions, which will be generically referred to as "drug-drug" interactions. These "drug-drug" interactions may result from more than one xenobiotic interacting with the same CYP450 isoform. One simple explanation for why such interactions can occur is shown for two chemical substances, D_1 and D_2, which react with the same subfamily of CYP450. If $K_1 >> K2$, then D_1 will be metabolized in preference to D_2, leaving unexpectedly high levels of unmetabolized D_2. A large number of drugs are recognized as inhibitors of specific subfamilies of CYP450. Thus, through this or similar mecha-

Table C-1. METABOLIC OXIDATION/REDUCTION REACTIONS

SUBSTRATE	ENZYME	PRODUCT	CHAPTER REFERENCE	OCCURRENCE
Alkane	CYP450	Alcohol	2	Uncommon
Alkene	CYP450	Peroxide	3	Uncommon
Aromatic ring	CYP450	Phenol	4	Common
Alcohol	ADH	Aldehyde/ketone	6	Common
Ether	CYP450	Phenol/ Aldehyde	8	Common
Aldehyde/ketone	ADH	1°/2° alcohol	9	Uncommon
Aldehyde	Aldehyde dehydrogenase	Carboxylic acid	9	Common
1° Amine	CYP450	Aldehyde	10	Common
2°/3° Amine	CYP450	1°/2° amine	10	Common
	FMO	Hydroxylamines		Common
3° Alkylamine	FMO	N-oxide		Common
Ester/amide/ carbonate/carbamate	Hydrolase	Carboxylic acid	12	
Thioether	CYP450	Sulfoxide/ Sulfone	14	Uncommon
	FMO	Sulfoxide/ Sulfone	14	Common
Thiol	FMO	Disulfide		Common

nisms of enzyme inhibition, a "drug-drug" interaction will occur. Another mechanism of "drug-drug" interaction occurs if a particular substance can induce an increase in activity of a specific CYP450 enzyme. This type of "drug-drug" interaction will lead to an unexpected decrease in the levels of a particular drug, thus reducing the biologic effectiveness of the drug (See *Foye's Principles of Medicinal Chemistry*, 5th ed., Chap. 8).

$$D_1 \xrightarrow[K_1]{CYP450} \overset{OH}{\overset{|}{D_1}}$$

$$D_2 \xrightarrow[K_2]{CYP450} \overset{OH}{\overset{|}{D_2}}$$

FLAVIN MONOOXYGENASE

Flavin monooxygenase (FMO) is a microsomal enzyme with a limited capacity to oxidize xenobiotic substrates. FMO oxidizes alkyl and aryl amines and thiols and thioethers. Tertiary alkylamines are oxidized to N-oxides, while secondary alkylamines, N,N-dialkylarylamines, and N-alkylarylamines form hydroxylamines.

$$R_1-\underset{\underset{R_3}{|}}{N}-R_2 \xrightarrow{FMO} R_1-\underset{\underset{R_3}{|}}{\overset{\overset{O}{\uparrow}}{N}}-R_2$$

(R_1, R_2, R_3 = alkyl)

$$R_1-\underset{\underset{H}{|}}{N}-R_2 \xrightarrow{FMO} R_1-\underset{\underset{OH}{|}}{N}-R_2$$

(R_1 = alkyl; R_2 = alkyl or aryl)

The oxidation of sulfur-containing drugs is confined to thiols, which are oxidized to disulfides, and thioethers, which are oxidized to sulfoxides or sulfones. While thioethers can also be oxidized via CYP450, in most cases this type of metabolism occurs through the intervention of FMO.

$$R-S-H \xrightarrow{FMO} R-S-S-R$$

$$R-S-R' \xrightarrow{FMO} R-\overset{\overset{O}{\uparrow}}{S}-R' \xrightarrow{FMO} R-\underset{\underset{O}{\downarrow}}{\overset{\overset{O}{\uparrow}}{S}}-R'$$

ALCOHOL DEHYDROGENASE

Alcohol dehydrogenase (ADH), a soluble enzyme found in the cytosol, is a nonhepatic enzyme capable of oxidizing primary and to a lesser extent secondary alcohols to aldehydes and ketones, respectively. While CYP450 is known to also have the ability of oxidizing selected alcohols to aldehydes, alcohol dehydrogenase appears to be the major alcohol-oxidizing enzyme. Alcohol dehydrogenase is also capable of reducing aldehydes and ketones to alcohols, although this does not appear to be as common a reaction.

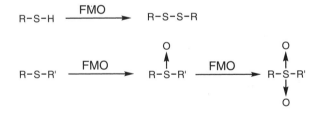

ALDEHYDE DEHYDROGENASE

There are a number of enzymes with the ability to catalyze the oxidation of an aldehyde to the corresponding carboxylic acid. Such enzymes are collectively categorized as aldehyde dehydrogenases. Included in this group is the enzyme ADH. These enzymes are commonly found in the cytoplasm.

Hydrolase Enzymes

Another collection of enzymes are those that generically may be called hydrolases. These enzymes attack the functional derivatives of carboxylic acids, leading to hydrolysis. Examples of such enzymes are carboxyesterases, arylesterases, cholinesterase, and serine endopeptidases. These enzymes are found in a wide variety of tissues and fluids. The hydrolase enzymes tend to be more effective in hydrolyzing esters than amides, but amidase enzymes do exist that break down amides to a carboxylic acid and an amine.

Amide hydrolysis tends to occur more commonly with highly lipophilic amides.

Conjugation Reactions

Phase 2 reactions consist of reactions in which new chemical bonds are formed between an organic functional group and a substrate such as glucuronic acid, sulfuric acid, acetic acid, or methyl groups. Generally, one thinks of a conjugation reaction as one that leads to metabolites with increased water solubility, but if one considers acetylation and methylation as conjugation reactions, it can be seen that water solubility may actually decrease. Also, it has been generally thought that conjugation of an organic functional group leads to loss of biologic activity, but recent examples have shown that in some cases the conjugates have increased activity. In most cases the conjugation reactions require the action of a cofactor to complete the reaction. The substrate and an endogenous molecule are brought together, leading to the formation of a new chemical bond. A phase 2 conjugation reaction can follow an initial phase 1 reaction, but it is not uncommon for a phase 2 reaction to occur as the only metabolic reaction. Also, it is possible that multiple conjugation reactions can occur to the same substrate, although this is unlikely since if the water solubility of the initial conjugation metabolite is high the product will be rapidly excreted, thus preventing further metabolism.

GLUCURONIDATION

Glucuronidation consists of the addition of D-glucuronic acid to a variety of substrates, including alcohols, phenols, primary and secondary amines, and carboxylic acids (Table C-2). The glucuronic acid is transferred to the substrate from the cofactor uridine-5′-diphoso-α-D-glucuronic acid (UDPGA). The enzyme responsible for catalyzing this reaction is a UDP-glucuronosyl transferase, which like the CYP450 represents a family of enzymes. These transferases are found in the endoplasmic reticulum of the liver and in epithelial cells of the intestine. As would be

Table C-2. METABOLIC CONJUGATION REACTIONS

CONJUGATION REACTION	SUBSTRATE	CHAPTER REFERENCE	OCCURRENCE
Glucuronidation			
	Alcohol	6	Common
	Phenol	7	Common
	1°/2°Amine	10	Common
	Carboxylic acid	11	Common
Sulfation			
	Alcohol	6	Common
	Phenol	7	Common
	1°/2°Amine	10	Uncommon
Acetylation			
	Arylamine	10	Common
	1°Alkylamine	10	Uncommon
Methylation			
	Alcohol	6	Common
	Phenol	7	Common
	Thiol		Common

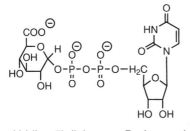

Uridine-5'-diphoso-α-D-glucuronic acid
(UDPGA)

R−X−H + UDPGA ⟶

(X = O, N,S, O-C)
      ‖
      O

Hydrophilic groups

Glucuronide

expected, glucuronidation will greatly improve water solubility of the metabolite through the presence of multiple alcohols and the carboxylic acid group present in the glucuronide. The latter group may be partially ionized at physiologic pH.

SULFATION

Sulfation consists of the addition of sulfuric acid to a variety of substrates, including alcohols, phenol, and to a lesser extent primary and secondary amines (see Table C-2). The sulfuric acid is transferred to the substrate from the cofactor 3'-phosphoadenosine-5'-phosphosulfate (PAPS). The enzymes responsible for catalyzing these reactions are again a family of transferases, the sulfotransferases. These transferases are found primarily in hepatic tissue. Water solubility of the sulfate conjugate is greatly increased since the sulfate is nearly completely ionized at physiologic pH.

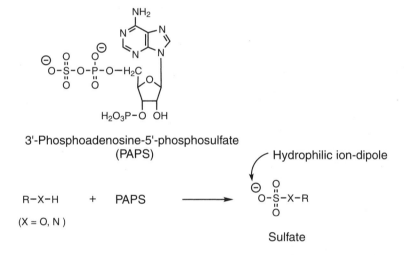

3'-Phosphoadenosine-5'-phosphosulfate
(PAPS)

Hydrophilic ion-dipole

$R-X-H$ + PAPS $\longrightarrow$

$(X = O, N)$

Sulfate

ACTYLATION

Acetylation consists of the addition of an acetate to primary aryl amines (common reaction) and to a lesser extent primary alkyl amines (see Table C-2). The acetate is transferred to the substrate from the cofactor acetylcoenzyme A (acetyl-CoA). The enzymes responsible for catalyzing these reactions are again a family of transferases, the N-acetyltransferases. These transferases are found primarily in hepatic tissue. Depending on the genetic makeup of the patient, the acetylation may be a fast reaction or a slow reaction. Slow acetylators will have higher blood levels of the substrate, while fast acetylators will have higher blood levels of the metabolite. Acetylation products usually show a decrease in water solubility.

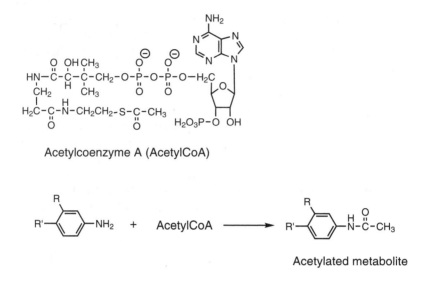

Acetylcoenzyme A (AcetylCoA)

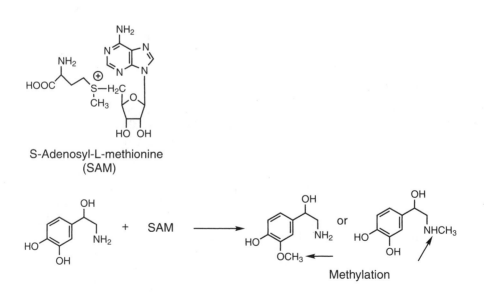

METHYLATION

Methylation consists of the addition of a methyl group to primarily alcohols, phenols, amines, and thiols (see Table C-2). The methyl is transferred to the substrate from the cofactor S-adenosyl-L-methionine (SAM). The enzymes responsible for catalyzing these reactions are again a family of O-, N-, and S-methyltransferases. Methylation products usually show a decrease in water solubility. Methylation reactions are quite common with endogenous substrates such as norepinephrine and dopamine and drugs that have structural similarities to the natural endogenous metabolites.

S-Adenosyl-L-methionine
(SAM)

Methylation

Index

Page numbers in italics indicate figures; those followed by t indicate tables.